'*Clearing the Fog* is a thoughtfu... ...th Long Covid. Dr Jackson draws on his own personal experiences with managing his mental health as well as the experiences of his patients to provide a guide on how to manage the challenges of Long Covid.'
– Dr Sanjay Gupta, author of *Keep Sharp*

'Dr Jackson expertly and compassionately explores the realities of Long Covid – from anxiety to brain fog – and reveals the actions we can take to support and empower ourselves and our loved ones. An essential guide for everyone touched by Long Covid.'
– Dr Mark Hyman, author of *Young Forever*

'Dr Jim Jackson, displaying his deep expertise and even deeper humanity, has produced a guide that provides a path forward for people living with Long Covid, and for many more managing other severe, chronic conditions. The sheer abundance of useful strategies is astonishing and conveyed in ways that are uplifting and encouraging. This book is sure to transform lives, enabling people to make meaningful progress despite dire health challenges.'
– Dr Harlan Krumholz, Director of the Center for Outcomes Research and Evaluation, Yale School of Medicine

'*Clearing the Fog* is full of invaluable – potentially life-saving – information and could be an indispensable handbook for millions of patients. Dr Jackson clearly lays out how to accept your illness, take steps to find specialist health providers or support services, and build a new life amid Long Covid. Following these steps may well save your career, your marriage, or your most deeply held dreams.'
– Ryan Prior, author of *The Long Haul*

'A timely and essential book. Jackson is a world-renowned expert on the effects of illness on cognitive functioning, and he seamlessly weaves together patient narratives, his own personal struggles, and cutting-edge research to create a uniquely empowering and insightful book. *Clearing the Fog* is not only for those suffering from Long Covid; it should be read by family members, by healthcare workers, by anyone who has been touched by this pandemic – which is, ultimately, all of us.'

– Daniela Lamas, author of *You Can Stop Humming Now*

'For two decades, I've witnessed my colleague, Dr Jim Jackson, expertly care for and support patients struggling with newly-acquired cognitive impairment and mental health difficulties after illness and into survivorship. His wisdom and empathy – on display throughout the pandemic in his treatment of patients with Long Covid – is distilled here on the pages of *Clearing the Fog*, a kind, profoundly human, and practical resource for long haulers, their families, and Health Care professionals. Grounded in science and guided by compassion, *Clearing the Fog* presents a way forward to the millions navigating Long Covid and other chronic illnesses, people who have been dismissed for far too long. Dr Jackson has listened to their concerns and provides solutions wherever possible and empathy when answers remain elusive. His book fulfills a driving unmet need in the literature and will bring hope to many.'

– Dr Wes Ely, author of *Every Deep-Drawn Breath*

CLEARING THE FOG

A Practical Guide to Surviving and Thriving with Long Covid

Dr James C. Jackson

Copyright © 2023 James C. Jackson

The right of James C. Jackson to be identified as the Author of the Work has been asserted by him in accordance with the Copyright, Designs and Patents Act 1988.

First published in the USA in 2023 by Little, Brown Spark an imprint of Hachette Book Group

First published in Great Britain in 2023 by Headline Home an imprint of Headline Publishing Group

First published in paperback in 2024

1

Cataloguing in Publication Data is available from the British Library

ISBN 978 1 0354 0191 8
e-ISBN 978 1 0354 0189 5

Offset in 10/14.6pt Bembo Book MT Std by Jouve (UK), Milton Keynes

Printed and bound in Great Britain by Clays Ltd, Elcograf S.p.A.

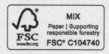

Headline's policy is to use papers that are natural, renewable and recyclable products and made from wood grown in well-managed forests and other controlled sources. The logging and manufacturing processes are expected to conform to the environmental regulations of the country of origin.

HEADLINE PUBLISHING GROUP
An Hachette UK Company
Carmelite House
50 Victoria Embankment
London EC4Y 0DZ

www.headline.co.uk
www.hachette.co.uk

To Michelle, who tends the garden of my heart and enriches
the world with faith, exuberance, and love.

Author's Note

First and foremost, this is a book about patients, real people whom I've been fortunate to know and who have courageously revealed their stories to me, both while thriving and while barely surviving. In every instance, they have been eager to share their personal journeys in the hope that they can help someone else who may be struggling. Out of an abundance of respect for the privacy of my patients, members of support groups, and those I consult with, I chose to create composite characters throughout the narrative, but while key details have been changed, they are all based in truth.

Further resources for patients and families can be found on the website for the Critical Illness, Brain Dysfunction, and Survivorship (CIBS) Center at www.icudelirium.org. We are an independently run, non-industry-funded educational resource, and we post all our resources free of charge.

Contents

CLEARING
THE FOG

Introduction:
Long Covid: An Epidemic

As the Covid-19 pandemic unfolded, the world watched in horror as grim tallies of daily death counts ticked steadily upward, reaching numbers that stunned us. The tragedy of lost lives cannot be overstated, but it obscured the fact that damage inflicted by the virus was measured not only in mortality rates but also in the unsettling persistence of debilitating symptoms long after the initial infection. Data emerged from numerous studies and clinical encounters with patients around the world showing that dying was not the only outcome to fear. On the contrary, long-term symptoms were present, and often life-shattering, in never-hospitalized individuals with "mild" disease as well as in those who had battled critical illness. These symptoms— more than two hundred have been recorded—are now universally known as long Covid and defined by the World Health Organization (WHO) as a syndrome "occurring in individuals with a history of probable or confirmed SARS-CoV-2 infection, usually three months from the onset of Covid-19, with symptoms that last for at least two months and cannot be explained by an alternative diagnosis."[1] This clinical definition, while useful, does not fully show the devastating impact that the condition can have on people and their loved ones as it turns their lives upside down. Estimates suggest that up to 200 million individuals around the world may be experiencing long Covid,[2] more than those with cancer and dementia combined.[3] If these individuals represented a country, it would be the eighth largest in the world[4] and, as variants continue to appear and disease spreads among populations, these numbers will only increase. Long Covid can affect cognitive, physical, and mental health functioning and occurs in many different demographics, including the young and the old, those from low, middle, and high socioeconomic circumstances, and from across a wide range of educational backgrounds. No one is immune.

Just a few months into the pandemic, I started a weekly support group for long Covid patients at the Critical Illness, Brain Dysfunction, and Survivorship (CIBS) Center in Nashville, Tennessee.[5] At first, we welcomed Covid survivors after an ICU stay, helping them to pick up the pieces of their lives after critical illness. Then, as we increased the number of support groups due to demand, we noticed a shift—many of our new attendees had never been admitted to a hospital. We began to realize how insidious this condition might be.

I was struck by the way our patients were battling both an illness and also the disbelief of the medical establishment. I had seen this happen over the years with survivors of critical illness who grapple with life-altering cognitive, psychological, and physical symptoms that prevent them from returning to the lives they once had. Their condition, known as post intensive care syndrome (PICS), has long been misunderstood and dismissed and patients often struggle in silence. I was determined to let my patients with long Covid know that they were heard and seen, and that treatments were available to them. Over time, it became clear that there were similarities between long Covid and other illnesses that occur after viruses such as myalgic encephalomyelitis/ chronic fatigue syndrome (ME/CFS), postural orthostatic tachycardia syndrome (POTS), and long Lyme disease. In fact, around half the people with long Covid are estimated to meet the criteria for ME/CFS.[6] Research into these conditions had already provided a knowledge base and I began to see that the way forward lay in collaboration and community, in using tried and true treatment methods while searching for new and creative approaches.

Susan tested positive for Covid after attending a bar mitzvah in early 2021 but experienced just a low-grade fever and a few days of malaise. Now, however, she is a Covid long hauler, as those with long Covid are often called, and grapples with cognitive problems so severe that they may end her career. A high-achieving attorney, she graduated from an Ivy League law school and vaulted to partnership status at a midsize urban law firm. Once renowned for always being on time and usually ten minutes early, she now routinely misses meetings if she remembers how to log on to them at all. She can no longer handle complex documents and makes errors drafting standard wills and contracts. Occasionally she forgets the names of clients whom she has worked with for years. For months, she has relied on her administrative assistant to run interference for her, but lately her deficits have become so obvious that there is no disguising them anymore. During a recent session of our support group, she told us, through tears, that in the days before she caught Covid, she had watched a news show about long haulers and scoffed at the specter of long Covid. She remembers saying under her breath that this illness might impact "weaklings" but not people like her. She added that she sleeps only fitfully now, worried about losing her job and how she will pay the mortgage on her spacious craftsman bungalow. Her old life—one she had worked hard to achieve—seems so distant, so unattainable. It's as if it belonged to somebody else.

Jose, another regular at our support group, is a grizzled former firefighter who switched to teaching middle school social studies a few years ago. He often reports that his brain is "working just fine" but it is cold comfort to him. This once fearless man used to run into burning buildings with a confidence that few of his fellow firefighters had seen before, but now he battles different demons—an unholy trinity of delusions, hallucinations, and depression—and on our Zoom calls he often sits at his desk, his attention far away, a vacant look on his face. Unlike Susan, he was profoundly ill with Covid, contracting it at a barber shop and rapidly "crashing" before waking up on a ventilator sixty-seven days after being admitted to a hospital in Mississippi. Disoriented and confused, he remembers little of the events that swirled around him over two long months, but one thing remains crystal clear in his mind—his graphic nightmares brimming with images of torture, rape, and carnage. He knows—on most days, at least—that these dreams cannot possibly be real but his recollections of them are visceral and vivid, and he often shares that these memories haunt him late at night, robbing him of any hope of sleep. His students, not knowing better, tease him when he falls asleep in class from exhaustion, and he agonizes about resigning from his job. Recently, when a balloon popped at a birthday party in the teachers' lounge, he almost jumped out of his skin, conjuring up reminders of his chronically anxious father, a Vietnam veteran whose mental health issues Jose once prayed he would never have to suffer. Post-traumatic stress disorder (PTSD), Jose tells us, is "supposed" to be a condition that impacts people after events such as war and sexual assault, but he's gradually embracing the idea that it visits survivors of Covid-19, too.

Zoey, a once-gregarious world traveler in her early forties who trekked across the Italian Alps the year before the onset of the pandemic, occupies a spot somewhere between her friends Susan and Jose. When she contracted Covid, she was sick enough to spend five days in the hospital but mercifully avoided the ICU. Yet this former college track athlete is so wracked by fatigue, anxiety, and discomfort that she rarely leaves her one-bedroom apartment. She's bewildered by the ways her body rebels against the commands she gives, and she has a hard time imagining, much less believing, that her life could ever be meaningful or rich. A newcomer to the group, she logs on to weekly Zoom calls, but while most of her peers are vertical, she is usually horizontal, lying on a bed or couch, or even stretched across the floor with her phone next to her head. Occasionally, when we talk about the value of processes like "acceptance," she crosses her arms and rolls her eyes, barely concealing her disgust for the idea that there might be value in making peace with a "new normal" that she can't abide. She has gone down a rabbit hole of speculative, unproven, and costly long Covid cures, spending money she can't afford, in a frantic effort to avoid a painful reality—that she may not get better at all.

At times optimistic and ebullient and at other times intensely sad, these survivors—in many respects the "lucky ones" as they have access to care—wrestle with cognitive problems ranging from humorous to concerning to life-threatening (putting a television remote control in the freezer, constantly forgetting to make mortgage payments, driving through red lights in crowded intersections, and nearly overdosing from taking the wrong medication), struggle with mental health challenges (intense health anxiety, depression, obsessive-compulsive disorder, PTSD, and suicidal thoughts), and sometimes battle fatigue so profound that a walk to the mailbox feels like a hike on the Appalachian Trail. They struggle under the weight of layers of guilt and shame, feel the pain of loneliness and isolation, and wish for the past lives to which they fear they will never return. They fight to maintain a modicum of hope as they see well-meaning physicians—both generalists and specialists—who shrug their shoulders and offer little guidance, meet with HR representatives at work who warn that they are approaching the limits of their time off or advise that their requests for long-term disability have been denied, and visit with family and friends who tell them they just need to "try harder and stop complaining" if they want to get better. Their stories are replicated millions of times over in long haulers in this country and around the world. Perhaps you see your own struggles reflected in their stories. Or maybe those of a family member, coworker, or friend. Exhausted by complex challenges, stung by the apathy of others, and confused by limited and often conflicting advice, people living with long Covid want to know they are seen and heard, and need guidelines on how to manage their illness and improve their functioning. In many ways, they are looking for hope.

Over the course of my many years of work as a psychologist helping patients to rebuild their lives after illness, I have been struck by the importance of my role as a guide—as someone who tries to meet my patients where they are in their lives, listens to their goals, communicates in ways that are accessible and relatable, creates a plan, and supports them in reaching it. I believe this is the most effective way to help my patients through these difficult times in their lives. In the early days of 2021, I became especially aware of the importance of guides for patients navigating illness when I struggled with my own mental health. Stoked by the challenges of the pandemic, my obsessive-compulsive disorder—previously well managed and under control—began raging, taking me to terrifying places I'd never visited. My guide was a clinical psychologist in a little stone cottage on Nashville's Music Row who helped me in transformative ways and to whom I often think I owe my life. She steadied me during hard days, gave me tools and fostered skills to help me face challenges, and outlined a vision for a brighter future and a road map for how to get there. On other occasions, I have found the steadying support of guides beyond the realms of illness: a mountaineer, a fitness coach, and, once or twice, an expert angler. Whether you are a long hauler yourself or are trying to support someone else, my goal in writing this book is to be your guide, helping you discover solutions, providing answers to your questions, and offering a path forward as you find your way through long Covid.

The chapters that follow address the primary concerns I have observed while engaging with long Covid patients and their families in clinical and research environments, during phone calls, in emails and social media conversations, and in consultations with colleagues. Namely, that a high percentage of patients feel that their brains don't work anymore, that they experience suffocating trauma and anxiety about the future, and that they feel as if they're stuck in an endless labyrinth as they seek treatment and resources. I have found that patients are happy to describe their priorities if only you ask them. This approach of empowering patients (and their families) to articulate what they perceive to be their problems, as opposed to doctors in starched white coats making these decisions, is known as patient-centeredness and is key to working with long Covid patients. Our patients are experts in their own condition, how it affects them, and what they need, and the values of patient-centered care inhabit every page of this book and inform my recommendations for patients and readers.

With a focus on cognitive impairments and mental health challenges—shown to exist in up to 50 percent of all long Covid patients[7]—my hope in writing *Clearing the Fog* is to offer support and information to help long haulers with many aspects of their new lives, from their first inklings that symptoms they are experiencing may be attributed to long Covid and beyond, as they seek and implement treatments. This is not an easy journey, and my aim is to accompany you, knowing that you may have felt discounted, shunned, and ignored at times by friends, family, and wide swaths of the medical establishment. Using my own experience with chronic illness, I offer suggestions on how to accept that life going forward may be different, not as a kind of resignation but as a foundation from which to build a new approach. In addition, I offer comprehensive, cutting-edge guidance, educating patients on the likely causes of long Covid and the complex scientific mechanisms that undergird it, as such knowledge is empowering. In this way, I hope to combat widely held misunderstandings about the condition, to demystify it, and take away some of its power.

I imagine that many people will come to this book looking for cures, for a way to get back to their pre-Covid lives. As I write, I am reminded of a story that my great-aunt Lurene, keeper of our family's genealogy, once told me about a distant relative of mine—Dr. R. V. Pierce, founder of the sprawling Invalids' Hospital and Surgical Institute in Buffalo, New York, and the most famous of the many turn-of-the-century hucksters who offered "snake oil" disguised as medicine to the masses. Positively Barnumesque, he convinced more than 2 million people to buy his thin paperback book, *The Common Sense Medical Advisor,* and sold even more bottles of his Golden Medical Discovery tonic—including one pristine example, slightly faded with the years, that sits on the mantle in my office. He preyed on people with late-nineteenth-century maladies who were desperately looking for a cure. Instead of a cure, Dr. Pierce offered a counterfeit, one unable to give relief despite hundreds of extravagant testimonies to the contrary contained in his many pamphlets. I am aware that many long haulers, just like my patient Zoey, are looking for a similar cure, a quick fix, perhaps, hoping for that one doctor who will finally understand them and their illness and launch them back to full health. While that route to healing may not be possible, I am able to offer multiple proven treatments and strategies that, over time, have helped many of my patients to see real improvement and transformation in their lives.

I offer evidence-based insights on how to address, treat, and manage cognitive dysfunction and mental health disorders, answering questions such as: When is it time to contact a specialist? What red flags might suggest that you or a family member is struggling with cognitive impairment? When is feeling sad a symptom of clinical depression? What treatments are available for my family member's cognitive impairment or exhaustion? My aim is to help long haulers and family members understand specific symptoms and conditions, know how and when to set up an evaluation, and be aware of different kinds of treatment options. These are complicated, often stressful processes, and having a guide to turn to can make a crucial difference.

In addition, I give information on navigating byzantine and often opaque healthcare systems that intimidate even sophisticated healthcare users, as I have seen the additional level of frustration they bring to my already exhausted patients. I offer practical guidance on whom to talk to—that is, advice on specialists to see, resources to pursue, and evaluations to consider as well as how to successfully engage in hard conversations with doctors, employers, and even family members. I find that having step-by-step advice to follow can ease such encounters, and I provide examples that can be used in many scenarios. In addition, you'll find practical information to assist in making decisions about returning to work, asking for work- and college-related disability accommodations or, alternatively, pursuing other options like short- and long-term disability. These everyday concerns are part of the new reality for many long haulers.

As someone who manages my own chronic illness, I am aware of and grateful for the support of my family. Long Covid is a condition that affects both the person with the condition and the people — usually family members and friends — who help them navigate their daily life. It was important to me to include a chapter that acknowledges this fact and provides tools and hands-on help for family members, too. According to research, family members experience rates of anxiety and PTSD comparable to those of patients[8,9] — their lives have changed irrevocably, too.

One day, while writing, I found myself listening to the radio playing in the background, and, as a child of the '80s, I immediately recognized the husky voice of Welsh songstress Bonnie Tyler amid a cascade of drums and piano riffs. Her iconic song "Holding Out for a Hero" from the movie *Footloose* was familiar to me, as were the song's lyrics that wondered why a "white knight upon a fiery steed" wasn't coming to save the day, and I thought about them through the lens of someone caring for long haulers. As was true of most diseases before the emergence of long Covid, such as cancer and Alzheimer's, there is no knight in shining armor, no breakthrough miracle cure, and, for that matter, no wizard with a magic wand who can cure every Covid-related ill with a whispered incantation. What there are, though, are strategies, treatments, and approaches that can make a substantial and, with time, even a dramatic difference in the lives of many people living with long Covid, leading to journeys of growth, recovery, and transformation. There are no shortcuts — but as poet Robert Frost said, "the best way out is always through." I feel privileged to accompany you on your journey of healing.

CHAPTER 1

WHERE TO BEGIN: A Road Map for Starting Your Long Covid Journey

For many people, long Covid begins with not feeling well in many different ways. Some may have experienced symptoms during a Covid-19 infection and, weeks later, are still struggling to improve. Others may have seemingly recovered from an initial bout of Covid but weeks or months later are beset with health problems again. Some may have spent time in an ICU and been discharged home, and yet they may not feel at all like themselves. And still others may have never known they had Covid at all, and yet now experience a multitude of physical, mental, or cognitive symptoms (or some combination of the three) that make it difficult to participate in life in ways they once had. There is no clear cause and no test for this ill-defined disease, and many people self-diagnose based on their experience of long-term effects that continue for weeks, months, and years after their initial Covid infection.

You, or someone you know, may have the feeling that something is wrong and that you're just not getting better, despite rest, or sheer strength of will, or the passage of time. Reluctant though you may be, it is time to turn to a healthcare professional.

Some of you may have come to this book because you have already been diagnosed with long Covid and, while you may not need advice on making a first appointment, the suggestions that follow are intended to be helpful for the first visit as well as for ongoing visits to other healthcare practitioners who may become part of your treatment plan.

For the first appointment, it is a good idea to see your primary care physician (PCP) or, if you live near one, to schedule a visit with a post-Covid clinic for an initial evaluation. (I go into more detail on these clinics on page 23.) Wait lists at post-Covid clinics are often long and you may need to wait several months for an initial evaluation. In this instance, it can make sense to schedule a post-Covid clinic appointment and, in the meantime, to see your primary care provider. I know the idea of making that first call or going online to set up an appointment can be daunting, as it may lead in a direction you're not ready to acknowledge. But making the call is key, and once you have gathered the courage to do so and made a note of the date in your calendar, it is a good idea to start planning for your visit.

PREPARING FOR YOUR APPOINTMENT

Many of my patients have told me how hard it was to get an initial doctor's appointment, especially at post-Covid clinics, and that, once booked, the visit took on mythic proportions, as if it held the key to the rest of their lives. This perspective, while understandable, is often unhelpful, as the diagnosis and treatment of issues related to long Covid is a process and rarely unfolds in a single encounter. Nevertheless, an initial appointment is critical and, while results can never be guaranteed, preparation is often the foundation for a successful outcome. This is especially true when symptoms of long Covid—such as cognitive dysfunction, anxiety, and exhaustion—threaten to undermine the appointment before the patient has even set foot in the doctor's office.

Recently, I met a patient with a diagnosis of mild cognitive impairment who was scheduled to see me at 9:30 in the morning. He arrived at the clinic thinking his appointment was at 7:30 and, by the time I saw him two hours later, he was frustrated, tired, and angry. Although we managed to work through these issues, they added to the stress of his already challenging day. In order to set yourself up for success at your first appointment, consider taking the following steps.

BEFORE YOUR VISIT

Think about this planning as a way to get the most out of your visit. You'll want to make sure that you arrive for your appointment on the right day, a little early if you can, with everything prepared and organized so that you can let your doctor know how your various symptoms impact your life, how your health has changed, and what you are hoping to address.

- Set reminders for the appointment on your calendars, phone, etc.
- Order or otherwise obtain any pertinent medical records if you are seeing a healthcare provider who doesn't have access to them. I've often had patients visit me who have received treatment at other hospitals, even in distant states such as Maine or California, and they haven't brought their medical records. This oversight makes it hard for even the best physician or diagnostician to have a full understanding of what is going on. Try to do this well in advance of your scheduled visit, as it may take some time for records to be accessed.
- Think about how you plan to travel to the appointment and how long it might take, and allocate ample travel time.
- If your appointment is not close to home, and if you have the resources, consider traveling the day or evening before to minimize the impact of time management problems prior to your visit.
- Ask a family member or friend to accompany you (I elaborate on this on page 28) and clarify how they can be most helpful during the visit. Do you want them to take notes, be an emotional support, or nudge you to ask questions you have forgotten? Make sure the appointment is on their calendar, too.

- Write up a brief history of your illness, including a timeline. Avoid long paragraphs and communicate simply with lists and bullet points. Your history *must* include details about your pre-Covid baseline level of functioning to help your healthcare practitioner better understand your current situation and how much you've declined. If you never had the ability to walk long distances and can't walk long distances now, you haven't appreciably declined. If you walked to the neighborhood park with your partner every evening after work and doing this now leaves you exhausted, your functioning has eroded. Similarly, if you used to finish a crossword puzzle every day and now can't get past the second clue, your cognitive functioning has changed. In the absence of accurate information about your usual capacities, your doctor may draw inaccurate conclusions that minimize the changes you are experiencing now.

- Keep a journal or notebook handy and track your symptoms, writing them down each day — or have someone help you do so. Make a note of when your symptoms occur and whether there seem to be any triggers.

- Keep note of your daily activities and how your symptoms affect you. Does unclear thinking make it difficult to drive, for example, or does it prevent you from speaking confidently during weekly team meetings at work? Are you too tired some days to get out of bed?

- Create a current medications list with details including medication name, dosage, and times it should be taken. Include vitamins and supplements on your list.

- Come up with a list of questions for the visit (see "Using a Script" on the next page as well as "During Your Visit" on page 19).

- Ask family and friends if there's anything you have missed that they think is important. Bear in mind that they may raise concerns about your functioning and/or highlight symptoms that you're not aware of. This can be hard to hear but try not to get angry or take it personally, and strive to receive their feedback in a nondefensive manner. Your loved ones are hoping to help and may have useful insights.

- Create a folder with all papers, forms, notes, etc., connected with the visit and make sure to take it with you. Include your journal or notebook and a pen for taking notes.
- Go through your folder before the visit to make sure the papers are labeled and organized for easy reference.

Using a Script

Sometimes it can be helpful to practice or role play a visit, especially if you are feeling anxious about it. The following script may be useful, allowing you to see what may be difficult for you to navigate. It highlights a few areas where patients often struggle — including the need to be specific in describing your symptoms, the importance of making sure *you* know exactly what your healthcare provider means and *they* know exactly what you mean, and the importance of being assertive in asking for the services you need — and it provides sample language that you could use at an appointment.

Clinician: Hi, Ms. Khoury, I'm Dr. Margolis. It's lovely to see you today. I'm glad we were able to get you on the schedule. I read your chart and it sounds like you've been struggling for a while.

Patient: I have. I'm having a really hard time after contracting Covid.

Clinician: What's going on?

Patient: All sorts of things, so many things, one struggle after the other.

Clinician: I'm so sorry. Can you tell me more?

Patient: Yes, my brain — it doesn't seem to be working as well as it did and I'm anxious a lot.

Clinician: These are very general concerns. Can you be more specific?

Patient: I think a lot about the eight days I spent in the ICU after getting sick with Covid. Every day I have disturbing memories of waking up in restraints and having no idea where I am. Honestly, I find myself ruminating about this experience all the time, and whenever something reminds me of it, my heart races and I feel panicked. And my memory—I've been having issues remembering the names of people close to me, and twice in the last week, I've forgotten to turn off the stove. I'm afraid that I might burn the house down if I keep this up.

Clinician: It sounds like you've got some neuropsychological issues in play.

Patient: Neuropsychological? I'm not sure what that means. Can you please clarify?

Clinician: Oh, yes, I'm using fancy terms. I meant to say that it sounds like you are dealing with memory problems and perhaps some mental health concerns. I see that you saw a psychologist at the hospital here a few years ago.

Patient: I did, yes, very helpful. But I want to clarify that the struggles I'm having are new and different. They're specific to my hospital stay, and they feel intense, not like general anxiety. I'm worried that I have PTSD after my hospital stay.

Clinician: I don't think you need to worry.

Patient: I am worried, I'm very worried. I know it's not your intention, but when you tell me not to worry, I feel sort of minimized and dismissed. Does that make sense? I would like a referral for a mental health professional, actually, a psychologist who can help me with these new concerns. Can you please give me such a referral?

Clinician: Thanks for telling me this. I'll contact our social worker and she will refer you. Now can you tell me more about what's going on with your memory?

In this example, the patient was able to name specific concerns and illustrate how they were impacting her life. She asked the doctor to clarify the meaning of "neuropsychological" and was able to reiterate that her symptoms were new when it seemed that the doctor was about to fold her concerns into an older diagnosis. When the doctor brushed aside her worry about her new symptoms, she stood her ground, politely and firmly, and advocated for a referral.

If, *before* the appointment, you can think about what you are hoping for from your visit, it will help you to navigate potential sticky areas while interacting with your doctor.

DURING YOUR VISIT

Your aim is to share the information you have prepared for your appointment, highlighting the most critical issues you would like to discuss, and to leave with a well-articulated plan of care. Bear in mind that many of the tasks described here are often best achieved if you are accompanied by someone who can take notes, nudge you to ask questions, and serve as your advocate. Most physicians welcome the involvement of such a person and if they are reluctant to do so, this may be a red flag. Here are ways to optimize your visit:

- Use your notes so you don't forget anything and try to be organized in your presentation.
- Tell your doctor your main symptoms, issues, and concerns, going through them one by one, with the most debilitating first. For example, "I'm exhausted all the time. I can't make it up the stairs and so I am sleeping on the couch."
- Answer the doctor's questions as succinctly as possible. Try not to get bogged down in small details.
- Share your medication list with your doctor.
- Listen carefully when the doctor explains their plan for next steps and if you don't understand anything, say so. Do not worry that you are bothering your doctor—you are there to receive their help and guidance, and they are there to give it.

- If your doctor does not seem to be planning for testing or follow-up, ask for clarification. (One to two follow-up visits with your doctor over twelve to fifteen weeks is standard in the treatment of most people with long Covid, so you almost certainly will have more than a single visit.) Your doctor may make referrals to specialists after the first visit or at a later time. If they don't— and you think a referral is important—seek to understand their reasoning and feel free to ask for one, if you believe it could be informative and helpful. If there are specific tests or experimental treatments that you think might help you, say so. If your doctor indicates that these are unnecessary or not appropriate, ask why.

- Clarify expectations about communication. Will the doctor reach out to you with test results, or will you be available to view them online? What kind of timeline should you expect? How is it best for you to get in touch with them after the visit?

- Ask about any clinical trials or research opportunities—either locally or nationally—that you may be eligible to participate in.

- Ask whether there is a social worker or case manager available who can help manage aspects of your care and assist in finding and accessing key resources.

- Query your doctor about their referral network. If you can have such a conversation before an initial visit, this is ideal but not always possible. Common questions might include: do they have close professional relationships with rheumatologists, immunologists, mental health professionals, cardiologists, and occupational therapists, just to name a few? Seeing such specialists is often a key building block in a comprehensive treatment plan, and access to a referral network is crucial. It is painful when help—in the form of a cardiologist who specializes in the treatment of postural orthostatic hypotension, for example, or a psychologist with expertise in PTSD—is available but cannot be accessed.

- Find out if your doctor will help you set up referrals. What about insurance preauthorization for testing or seeing specialists? Is that your responsibility?
- Is your doctor willing to provide support by completing paperwork related to job or school disability accommodations, disability insurance, or workers' compensation? Are they willing to advocate for you? Do they seem personally invested in this? Is it seen as part of their job? Patients have told me that some healthcare providers charge quite high fees for such services, so make sure you are well informed.
- Before you leave your appointment, check in with yourself. Stop, think, and reassess. Are you feeling confused or dismissed? Does it seem as if there are questions that haven't been answered? Now is the time to ask them, or say you're unclear. Your family member or friend, if one has accompanied you, can be invaluable here and can ask anything that doesn't seem to have been covered.
- Ask for an appointment summary that describes concisely what was discussed and concluded and sets out planned next steps. This typically cannot be provided at the time but could be given to you after the visit, usually within seven to ten days.
- If your doctor, or a member of their team, gives you paperwork or appointment cards, make sure you put them into your folder immediately—or take a photo of them on your phone, if you can.

After your appointment, if you have the time and energy, it can be helpful to take a moment to recharge, maybe to hydrate and have something to eat. The visit will probably have drained you physically and emotionally. If someone came with you, you could debrief while the visit is fresh in your minds but plan to go over the details with them or alone later that day or the next. Resist the tendency to second-guess yourself and worry that you should have detailed your symptoms a little more clearly or been a bit more explicit in describing your history.

Practice self-compassion, realizing that you probably did a good job and will have other opportunities to tell your story.

AFTER YOUR VISIT

There will likely be a variety of key tasks to attend to after your initial visit. It can be useful—and quicker—to enlist someone to help you so that your to-do list doesn't feel overwhelming. Follow-up items may include:

- Making a note in your calendar to follow up with your doctor about test results from your initial visit, if you are expecting any.
- Making appointments for testing or with specialists, as recommended and referred by your doctor.
- Keeping records of these appointments in one location or, for example, in an online calendar and, if possible, setting alerts and reminders. I've had many patients write appointment times on scraps of paper (I've done this many times myself) or even on their hand—don't do this!
- Making sure that someone else is aware of your appointment schedule.
- Filling prescriptions that your doctor may have given you and updating your medications list. If you have many different medications, get yourself a pill organizer. There are a variety of excellent ones to choose from.
- Following your doctor's instructions as closely as possible. These could include recommendations about diet, exercise, driving long distances, and not over-exerting yourself.
- Notifying your doctor of any new symptoms or changes to old ones and continuing to fill out your symptom tracker so you have a written reminder of all symptoms to share during a future visit.

In an ideal world, visits to healthcare practitioners go according to plan and result in a deeply satisfying partnership where issues are addressed, referrals are made, problems are resolved, and symptoms are managed. In the real world, especially with long Covid, things don't always unfold this way. The process isn't tidy, is rarely linear, can be slow, and can involve several trips down a blind alley on a road to greater understanding and, ultimately, progress. This is, in part, because long Covid remains a relatively new syndrome and can be challenging to healthcare workers who are unfamiliar with its many nuances and expressions. Sometimes primary care doctors are uninformed, overwhelmed by large caseloads that make personalized care difficult, and attribute medical problems to psychological causes in ways that are unhelpful.

If you feel that you are not being heard or taken seriously by your doctor, or that they are out of their depth and lack relevant expertise, or are reluctant to make referrals, an effective option—as described earlier in the chapter—is to go to a post-Covid or long Covid clinic. These one-stop shops are led by an interdisciplinary team of healthcare providers who specialize in the care and management of patients battling the lingering effects of Covid. At the time of this writing, 297 such clinics exist in the United States, with many more around the world, and their number is growing.[1] If your primary care provider doesn't know of one, you can easily find one via an online search for "post-Covid clinic" or "long Covid clinic." Their specialized services vary from center to center but often include a comprehensive array of diagnostic tests or workups, opportunities to participate in experimental therapies or clinical trials, access to experts from typically hard-to-find specialties such as neuroimmunology or integrative medicine, and clinicians who have had significant experience working with complex cases of long Covid, enabling them to more quickly get to the heart of the matter. It is often in these clinics where patients receive a diagnosis of long Covid for the first time, or one of many diagnoses that are deemed a Post-Covid Condition such as postural orthostatic tachycardia syndrome, a disorder of the autonomic nervous system, or myocarditis, inflammation of the heart muscle.

COMMUNICATING WITH YOUR
HEALTHCARE PRACTITIONER

It's important to note that when you have a conversation with your healthcare provider—whether before, during, or after your visit—you always have the right to ask as many questions as you want. These might include questions about a provider's philosophy of care, or their views on long Covid, including whether they have had Covid themselves, or about your care plan. If you have doubts about their answers, consider raising these misgivings, and remember that differences of opinion, and even conflict, can be healthy and constructive as long as you feel that you are on the same page. Brushing concerns aside, while often an effective way to avoid tension in the moment, is rarely a successful long-term strategy. If your worries are of a nature that can't be resolved, consider finding another provider. Patients are typically reluctant to do this but speaking from experience, I prefer it—in my practice, if you are unhappy with my care or have decided that we are not an effective fit I want to know that, and I want to help you find a provider who may be better for you. Most physicians feel the same way.

As an aside, if you find yourself feeling frustrated by your doctor or offended by a comment they made, consider taking a minute to make sure you've correctly understood where they are coming from. Many years ago, I did a sabbatical in the United Kingdom, where I studied cognitive rehabilitation at a treatment center in a sleepy little hamlet outside of Cambridge. I loved my time there, but I particularly missed the delicious Southern barbecue that is a passion of mine. One weekend we were in Trafalgar Square in London, and I saw a sign in the distance. It appeared to say "Barbeque Festival" and although I thought this was odd, my interest was piqued. My heart sank when, on closer inspection, it said "Baroque Festival." As a famous sage once said, "Don't believe everything you think."

RECEIVING A DIAGNOSIS

Receiving a diagnosis of long Covid from your healthcare provider—or post-acute sequelae SARS-CoV-2 infection, as it is also called—can be a straightforward process for some and more complicated for others. If the difficulties you are experiencing months after contracting the Covid-19 virus did not previously exist, are well defined, and cannot be better explained by other factors, then they probably reflect long Covid. If, however, the symptoms are subtle and may have previously been present in some form (e.g., a patient with multiple sclerosis with a long history of waxing and waning fatigue reports feeling "pretty worn out" weeks after their Covid infection), determining whether they are due to long Covid is challenging. In addition, many conditions that emerge after contracting Covid present in atypical ways or as normal on standard tests, making them difficult to diagnose. Despite these challenges, accurate diagnoses can usually be made over time when age-old principles of clinical medicine (such as physical examinations, exhaustive history taking, and careful listening to patients and families) are utilized in concert with results from diagnostic testing.

A diagnosis is not the end of the road. Far from it. Instead, it is the beginning of the next part of the journey. As a general rule, receiving a diagnosis can be difficult and upsetting, and patients and their families experience it in vastly different ways. Over the last twenty years, I've performed thousands of diagnostic evaluations of veterans at our local VA hospital, and I've noticed that upon learning that they have PTSD, to name just one example, some of them cry tears of joy, relieved that their problem has a name and has finally been acknowledged. Others are horrified, believing that they are "damaged goods," their new diagnosis a giant scarlet letter that they're destined to wear around their neck like a millstone. Having a healthcare provider lean in and gently say, "I think you have long Covid" or an array of post-Covid conditions evokes similar reactions. For some, it is a welcome answer to a mystery that helps explain why they put their car keys in the refrigerator, battle with balance, or bend under the weight of crushing fatigue. For others, it is a source of great shame, and, unfortunately, an opportunity for self-blame. Many of my patients with lingering issues ruminate over the fact that they went to a birthday party, a work conference, or a hair salon and caught Covid and criticize themselves harshly, telling themselves that if they had only been more fastidious or used better judgment, they wouldn't have symptoms of long Covid today. For others—perhaps most of the patients I see—a diagnosis is confirmation of their worst fears. They believe the bright future they once imagined may be unattainable now, that their life journey may be irrevocably changed. This moment of knowing is pivotal, fundamental, and likely hard. It is a crucial step for you, and for your family members, and taking in this news that you have an illness that affects many, if not all, aspects of your life can be overwhelming. You may feel anger, sadness, fear, relief, numbness, and myriad other emotions, as you realize you have a new normal to contend with. This is to be expected and it's okay to express these feelings.

In recent years, I've experienced my own new normal, a chronic condition that I don't want, that I didn't ask for, and that I'm learning to live with every day. I have obsessive-compulsive disorder (OCD). Not the charming version that people joke about that results in perfectly folded napkins, sparkling countertops, and exquisitely organized closets. No! Like millions of others with OCD around the world, my chronic malady is far from benign, generating twisted thoughts and fears that are sometimes primal and all-consuming. Such as worries that I will lose control of my car and run over the man who directs traffic at the crosswalk I drive through every day, thoughts that I might have robbed a bank (or two or three) in the distant past and that the police will be arriving at my house to arrest me sometime soon, or beliefs that I had impregnated a close friend even though we had never been remotely intimate. These are the types of symptoms that started emerging several years ago and led me to a psychologist, knowing there was something wrong that I hoped could be fixed.

For a long time, we searched for a diagnosis. We explored the usual suspects over a number of months — anxiety and PTSD — before moving on to other possibilities, including psychosis, but nothing seemed to explain my symptoms or help me with them. Finally, we landed on a chronic psychiatric condition that accounted for my many challenges. Though I had desperately wanted a diagnosis, upon learning that I had OCD, I felt utterly broken, bewildered, and ashamed. This wasn't supposed to happen to me — I was a psychologist, and I had carefully cultivated the garden of my mental health for decades, wrongly believing, at least unconsciously, that this would insulate me against pathologies of various kinds.

I told my psychologist that we needed to eradicate my OCD because with it, I — and my life going forward — could not possibly be okay. To my profound dismay, my psychologist didn't play along. She didn't offer any greeting-card slogans, tiresome bromides, or platitudes, but instead calmly introduced a few realities. She gently told me that I had a chronic illness, one that could likely be effectively managed (while acknowledging there were no guarantees) but wouldn't disappear anytime soon despite my best efforts at wishing it away or scouring the internet looking for miraculous cures.

With this diagnosis, I was looking at a new normal that I had to reckon with and find a way to fold into my life. I had a choice — I could deny it or try to accept it. As I contemplated my decision, I remembered my tendency to kick the can down the road while avoiding hard truths that demanded a response. I recalled a day, decades earlier, when the check engine light came on in my trusty white Mazda and I covered it with a sticky note and kept on driving. A few short weeks later, my car gave up the ghost on the side of the road on a humid Tennessee evening. As I waited for the tow truck, I wished I had not been so avoidant.

In many ways, as you grapple with your new normal of long Covid, you have a similar reality in front of you, one that demands you accept that your brain and body are not working as they once did, asks you to respect new limitations, and calibrate accordingly while knowing that this acceptance is not a kind of giving up. Instead, it is a base, a foundation from which to navigate your new situation, to find treatments and resources, and to manage your condition as effectively as possible.

SUPPORT SYSTEMS

The value of a good support system is often underappreciated until you need it, and nowhere is this truer than in the case of long Covid. When I look at the many patients I interact with, whether in our research studies, or in my clinic, I've noticed that those who have more support tend to do better. Some are blessed with large and nurturing networks such as tight-knit extended families, caring neighbors, longtime work colleagues, or friends from the Rotary Club or from faith communities, and they can more readily leverage support for themselves when illness strikes. Even in such situations, however, people are often slow to respond unless they are aware of your needs. Against this backdrop, learning to ask effectively for support is crucial, especially because data from social science research suggest that most humans are eager to answer the bell when called upon. To be most successful in your requests for help, follow these guidelines:

- Communicate your needs clearly and specifically. (For example, "Can you drive me to my cardiology appointment next Tuesday at ten a.m.? It is eighty miles away in Ann Arbor. I am exhausted, and I don't believe I can drive that far.")
- Whenever possible, ask for assistance ideally in person or, if not, by phone. Asking for help via email is less effective. Research has

demonstrated that requests for help made during face-to-face encounters are up to thirty-four times more likely to succeed than requests for help made via email.[2]

- Don't be afraid of inconveniencing people. Frequently we reject overtures of help because we worry about imposing. When someone offers help, assume they are operating in good faith, even if it is potentially challenging for them, and accept!

Nearly thirty years ago, my wife, Michelle, and I moved to Los Angeles to attend graduate school. We had left behind family and friends in Kalamazoo, Michigan, and we felt intensely lonely and unmoored. We hoped to find friends at a nearby church and each Sunday we made our way there, believing that this would be the day when we'd be embraced by people who had been waiting for us their entire lives. It never happened. One morning, while feeling especially discouraged, I stood up in our little Sunday school class and announced that we were flailing. As Michelle sat beside me crying, I talked about the isolation we felt, and made a plaintive request for help. This was decades before Brené Brown made vulnerability acceptable, when appearing needy was an unforgivable sin, especially for people, like me, invested in being perceived as competent and capable. When we arrived home later that day, our answering machine held more than a dozen messages—requests to go to the movies, to come over for dinner, to share life. The support we received from our newfound friends in the months and years that followed transformed our lives, saved our marriage, and altered the course of our future.

Among your friends and family members, you may find that different people are good at providing different kinds of support. If possible, you should try to assign people to the various types of help you may need. One friend may be excellent at coordinating your medical records and paperwork but less comfortable in offering a shoulder to cry on.

Emotional Support

Sometimes you may want to talk with someone about how you feel, about your emotional response to your illness, your capabilities, and your limitations. Within your network of people, you'll want to identify someone (or several people), if possible, who is at ease with listening to you and validating you, without necessarily jumping in to fix anything. If you feel you need additional — or confidential — emotional support, you may consider talking with a trained professional such as a mental health practitioner or social worker. I provide more details on mental health specialists in Chapters 4 and 5.

Informational Support

You may appreciate help in navigating the flood of paperwork, appointments, and logistics that may accompany your diagnosis. Ask someone to assist you with such tasks as organizing your calendar, making medical appointments, handling health and disability insurance forms, and following up on prescription refills. It is easier, if possible, to tackle these jobs in small increments of time, with assistance, before they pile up and becoming overwhelming.

Medical Support

Your medical support system, namely a community of medical providers who act in ways that reflect empathy and respect and who align with your needs and values, is crucial on your journey. While ivory tower pedigrees can be proof of expertise, they are of little practical value if the physicians possessing them don't return your calls or emails, prioritize your care, or display a consistent willingness to go the extra mile in treating your various conditions. When choosing members of your medical support system, look for expertise combined with the attributes that cause you to feel heard and understood. It can be hard to know if this is the case before a visit, so asking for recommendations and referrals can be important, as can paying some attention to online reviews. Find competent providers who care for you deeply and you will generally be well served.

You may also need a medical support person or two among your family members or friends, someone who can help you make sense of your interactions with doctors and your medical test results and can even stay informed on recent research findings on long Covid.

Support Groups

Currently I lead three long Covid support groups weekly—two for patients and one for families—as well as a weekly support group for survivors of critical illness that includes many patients who were hospitalized due to Covid. Such groups, long relied on as literal lifelines for certain patient populations, have proliferated during the pandemic and exist in both in-person and online contexts. They typically are available at no cost, and, in the words of many patients, can be one of the single most valuable aspects of long Covid treatment. I elaborate further on the benefits of support groups in Chapter 8.

We've covered a lot of ground in this chapter and, as I'm writing on the first day of summer, I'm reminded of times as a boy when twenty or thirty of us piled into an old yellow bus and went to the beach at Lake Michigan for the day. We were usually hot and sticky by the time we arrived from sitting on black vinyl seats, and a few of us would run down the steep dunes and straight into the water. But not me. I still remember how cold the water felt, frigid even in July or August, and I was usually reluctant to jump in, hanging back on the beach. But once in, I never regretted it.

The first step is always difficult to take. You may still be standing on the shore, not wanting to make that initial appointment or to move beyond being given a diagnosis. But I believe that if you make the decision to find out more, you'll be better able to move forward, face the future, no matter how uncertain it may feel, and start to find some answers.

CHAPTER 2

COGNITIVE IMPAIRMENT IN LONG HAULERS: More Brain Injury Than Brain Fog

When American inventor Thomas Edison said, "The chief function of the body is to carry the brain around," he was perhaps not completely wrong. At the very least, his insight underscores a reality that we all understand—the brain is vital to our well-being and its preservation is a priority. Since early in the pandemic, cognitive impairment, or "brain fog," has been one of the most widely reported difficulties for people with long Covid. In this chapter I'll look at how it can impact and disrupt lives, show the ways it might manifest in daily living, and provide recommendations for when and how to set up a visit to a specialist for an evaluation.

The term *brain fog* has long been used in medical and nonmedical literature to describe cognitive impairment in various conditions such as cancer, lupus, multiple sclerosis, HIV, fibromyalgia, and myalgic encephalomyelitis/chronic fatigue syndrome. The term may seem apt as it expresses the lack of clarity and sluggishness in thinking that people feel as they struggle with concentration, memory, confusion, fuzzy thoughts, and mental fatigue, but it can also have the effect of minimizing the debilitating impacts that often accompany it. I'll refer to brain fog as cognitive impairment throughout the book in order to highlight its seriousness—the brain has suffered an injury—and the fact that many long haulers have had their lives turned upside down by it.

In a 2021 study conducted by my Emory University colleague, Abeed Sarker, he and his team extracted and analyzed data from more than 42,000 posts by more than 4,000 Reddit users in a long Covid forum in order to discover symptoms self-reported by users.[1] Sarker found that approximately one in three individuals (32.8 percent) expressed difficulties of a cognitive nature long after the resolution of their acute Covid symptoms. The findings of this innovative investigation have been—and continue to be—backed up consistently by other studies. An analysis of almost two hundred survivors of Covid-19 and a similar number of controls,[2] published in two papers in *Frontiers in Aging Neuroscience* in June 2022, showed that 78 percent of those who had contracted Covid reported having cognitive problems months after the onset of their illness, with particular problems in areas of concentration, sluggish thinking, forgetfulness, and word finding.[3] Along with these self-reported difficulties, problems across a range of cognitive domains were observed on neuropsychological tests, and more cognitive impairment was seen in the Covid survivors. Multiple other studies and investigations have reached similar conclusions.

Research by Gwenaëlle Douaud and her team at Oxford University, published in a landmark paper in *Nature* in 2022, highlighted this extraordinary truth: patients' brains change in observable ways after contracting Covid-19—and in some cases patients had lost up to 2 percent of their brain tissue.[4] Using cutting-edge neuroimaging modalities that evaluate brain structure and neuronal interconnections, Douaud observed brain damage in a significant number of patients, including those who were never hospitalized for Covid and those who experienced mild illness. In cognitive functioning tests, given as part of the study, participants who had previously contracted Covid displayed specific deficits in processing speed, meaning that they performed complex tasks slowly. These findings were a surprise to virtually everyone except, perhaps, the community of long haulers living with post-Covid cognitive impairment.

In another study, world-renowned brain-injury researcher Dr. David Menon worked with a cohort of nearly fifty survivors of Covid-associated critical illness treated at one of England's leading medical centers.[5] Comparing them to more than four hundred control patients, he found that up to 76 percent of patients had significant cognitive deficits six months after their hospital discharge, reflected in slow and error-filled performances on a battery of cognitive tests. Survivors scored especially low on tasks such as verbal analogical reasoning, a result that supports the often-reported difficulty that long haulers experience in finding words. Most concerning, they displayed a degree of cognitive decline equivalent to that which occurs between the ages of fifty and seventy, a loss of ten IQ points.

While the evidence strongly supports the fact that Covid cases can lead to persistent cognitive symptoms, it's important to note that cognitive problems seen in long haulers are not usually consistent with those associated with Alzheimer's disease and dementia more generally, which are characterized by memory loss (of facts, important dates, and personal experiences).[6] In addition, post-Covid cognitive decline is not typically progressive in nature, and the memory deficits do not seem to degrade over time, an enormous relief to many long haulers.[7] As Dr. Menon noted, "Cognitive impairment is common to a wide range of neurological disorders, including dementia, and even routine aging, but the patterns we saw—the cognitive 'fingerprint' of COVID-19—was distinct from all of these."

We've known for decades that various medical conditions, including viral infections, can and do contribute to cognitive problems. We have seen this happen with Zika,[8] Ebola,[9] SARS,[10] Epstein-Barr, West Nile, and other diseases, and it is well documented in scientific literature.[11] A few years ago, I saw the effects of the Dengue virus on the brain when Felix, a herpetologist (a specialist in reptiles and amphibians), came to see me at the ICU Recovery Center at Vanderbilt from his home in California after contracting the disease on a trip to the rain forest in Nicaragua. He had developed encephalitis (inflammation of the brain) and displayed severe memory issues as well as problems with attention and concentration. He frequently forgot the names of colleagues, especially those he had just met, and struggled to keep track of his notes and research materials. Questions remain about the specific mechanisms that contribute to cognitive impairment in people with long Covid though research continues in the laboratory, in animal models, and in clinical investigations.[12] These mechanisms vary to a degree across populations and may be different in those who were hospitalized or in the ICU due to Covid and those who had mild acute symptoms.[13] For people who were hospitalized, possible causes or contributors include direct effects of infection on the brain, hypoxia (inadequate oxygen supply), multiple organ dysfunction, delirium, and the development of a "leaky" blood–brain barrier, which can lead to harm to or death of brain cells. For other long haulers, possible contributors include direct effects on the brain as well as an overactive immune response, which can impede the brain's neural connections, and neuroinflammation, which can contribute to the dysregulation and degradation of neuronal cells.

The research on long Covid that is emerging from medical trials and investigations and published in prestigious academic journals describes the experience of thousands of patients through figures, graphs, and mean and median scores. But in my clinic and support groups, and in others around the world, we see what these data represent in our patients' daily lives as they deal with the frustrating reality of brain dysfunction. You, too, may know firsthand the ramifications of living with cognitive impairment.

MEGAN'S STORY

Forty-year-old Megan came to my clinic after learning about our work with long Covid survivors from the local news. A lifelong high achiever, she was on the cusp of completing a master's degree in computer science when, in March 2021, she contracted Covid-19. She navigated her illness at home and thought the worst was behind her until she noticed an array of cognitive problems that hindered her progress on her master's thesis. Her data collection was mostly complete, but she found that she just couldn't write it up, no matter how hard she tried. Even when she was able to motivate herself and find the energy to sit at her desk, she couldn't focus on her work, finding her attention often straying elsewhere. For weeks, she vowed to herself that she would do a better job the next day, but as each new day came and went she realized that she was never going to be able to finish the paper. She was devastated.

At the same time, Megan was working a few days a week at an engineering company. Once a respected performer there, she started hiding in the shadows, afraid that interactions with others would expose the problems she was having remembering names and conversations. She frequently forgot about meetings and stumbled through those that she did attend, often unable to follow the details of projects and lost for words when called upon to clarify a point. At first, her well-deserved reputation for excellence insulated her performance from scrutiny, but eventually her manager concluded that her deficits were too pervasive and severe to ignore. In the end, she chose to leave her job, preferring that option to being fired, but even so, she was stunned to find herself on the disability rolls, her life in disarray.

When I first encountered Megan, I was struck by the dramatic change that had occurred in her life in such a short period of time. As was she. The word *surreal* peppered our conversations and she described being in a perpetual state of shock. She was trying to understand her options and hoping to chart a path toward healing and recovery. I imagined that this multifaceted task seemed as daunting, if not more so, than one of her engineering projects.

Megan's story is both unique in its details and yet similar in its broad strokes to that of many of my other patients—and to countless other Covid survivors around the world. Although the particulars may be different, perhaps you recognize yourself or a family member in her struggles. Maybe you were working, going to school, keeping house, raising your children, or easing into a well-deserved retirement, when your life was upended by Covid-19's effects on the way your brain works. It is not an easy situation to be in.

In caring for patients such as Megan, I have found that they can suffer from a sense of being overwhelmed, believing that their brain— and themselves along with it—is completely broken. The British philosopher and father of the scientific method, Sir Francis Bacon, once said that "knowledge itself is power," and I have seen this to be the case with Covid long haulers. The more they understand the mechanics of the difficulties they are experiencing, the more empowered they feel— and the more able to see the possibility of a way forward with a treatment plan.

To this end, in the next section I provide an overview of different kinds of cognitive functioning and highlight ways that cognitive impairment may occur and undermine a person's ability to carry out what were once routine tasks.

SIX KEY DOMAINS OF COGNITIVE FUNCTION

The *Diagnostic and Statistical Manual of Mental Disorders*, Fifth Edition (*DSM-5*), defines six key domains of cognitive function, with each having various sub-domains.[14] I find it helpful to use these six in my work with patients, including long haulers. Other healthcare professionals may prefer to focus on a greater or fewer number of domains, and considerable disagreement exists among experts about what components each domain comprises. The six neurocognitive domains that I use, listed in alphabetical order, are attention, executive functioning, language, memory, perceptual motor function, and social cognition.

Attention

This domain encompasses four broad components: selective attention, sustained attention, divided attention, and processing speed. *Selective attention* refers to the ability to choose which information in a particular situation to attend to and which to ignore, while *sustained attention* is the capacity to pay attention over a prolonged period, and *divided attention* is the ability to process more than one piece of information at a time. Problems with attention can manifest in different ways, including not being able to focus on a conversation in a noisy room or listen to directions while looking at your phone, being easily distracted, and having problems engaging in tasks — even enjoyable ones such as playing a board game or baking a cake — in a concentrated manner. My patient Megan's thesis writing was doomed by cognitive deficits in the attention domain.

During a recent long Covid support group session, one of our patients with pronounced attention problems mentioned that she had backed into her brother's car in the driveway on Thanksgiving as she was thinking about something else. In response, another member of the group, a traveling salesman who logs many highway miles each week, confided that he had recently driven through a red light, narrowly avoiding a car wreck. "I wasn't paying attention," he said. "My mind was on the news on the radio."

Processing speed refers to the amount of time it takes someone to identify, process, and respond to information, and deficits in this ability appear to be especially common in those with long Covid. It includes both "active" (consciously attentive) and "automatic" activities — those you usually engage in without thinking, such as putting the key in the ignition before driving or grabbing a cart in the grocery store. As with attention, processing speed is foundational to many cognitive abilities, and impairment in this area contributes to problems in other areas of cognitive functioning as well. Numerous studies suggest that processing speed deficits are the primary cognitive problem experienced by long haulers.[15,16,17] In one such study, investigators from Italy followed thirty-seven survivors of Covid-19, ranging in age from twenty-two to seventy-four, and evaluated them approximately six months after hospital discharge (none spent time in the ICU).[18] While 26 percent had problems with memory, nearly 1 in 2 (42 percent) displayed deficits in processing speed, a finding consistent with what my colleagues and I see in our patients.

These impairments often show up in striking delays in the time it takes someone to respond to questions, including those posed in routine conversations or meetings. One of my patients became reluctant to give presentations, a key feature in his sales and marketing job, knowing that he would have to think on his feet in answering questions. It had always been one of his strengths and yet, since developing Covid-19, he found himself searching for answers and struggling to formulate responses in a timely fashion to even the most rudimentary of queries. Slower processing speed can also mean taking much longer in getting through work- or school-related assignments, something that can become exacerbated if there are many different parts to a project. My patient Megan struggled with this, finding it difficult to get individual tasks done on time until entire projects fell way behind schedule.

Executive Functioning

Executive functioning (EF) refers to a range of abilities involved in the coordination of cognition, including planning, decision-making, inhibition (the ability to limit or restrain an impulse or an action), mental flexibility, response to feedback, and working memory. In general, these terms are self-explanatory, but *working memory* may be unfamiliar to some readers. It skirts the boundary between EF and memory and refers to the process of holding on to small pieces of information to complete immediate cognitive tasks, e.g., remembering an email address while you type it or getting directions to a friend's house and retaining them until you arrive there. When people display deficits in executive functioning, they often find it difficult to manage their behavior in ways that accomplish long-term goals, making it hard to function effectively in social, academic, and work roles, particularly if these roles are at all demanding. Research has demonstrated that problems with EF, which causes executive *dys*function (ExD), are associated with difficulties in areas such as driving,[19,20] handling finances,[21,22] managing medication, and navigating healthcare systems.[23]

Sometimes people with ExD develop idiosyncratic workarounds that can be both inefficient and fraught with risk. One of my patients came up with his own system for taking about twenty different medications a day as he was overwhelmed by the idea of setting up and keeping to a pill schedule. Instead of taking them as prescribed, he put one of each pill in a bottle every morning and swallowed them all together with a glass of water. One day, he came home from the pharmacy with a prescription for Warfarin, a potentially lethal blood thinner and, in a rush and distracted by an episode of his favorite television show, *Wheel of Fortune,* he inadvertently swallowed the full bottle of thirty Warfarin pills, thinking he was taking the bottle filled with his daily supply. He spent a week in the hospital undergoing observation due to concerns about a cerebral hemorrhage.

Language

In the language domain, we include the ability to find words, use grammar and syntax, and name objects as well as receptive and expressive capabilities (listening and talking) and verbal fluency. The latter refers to the retrieval of information from memory, e.g., How many words can you name that start with the letter *L*? How many fruits and vegetables can you think of? Cognitive impairment in the language domain can have immediate and impactful consequences because it limits and impedes communication, which is central to effective functioning.

Many of my long Covid patients struggle with naming objects. This can occur in several ways. *Semantic paraphasias* are speech errors in which the word a person uses may be incorrect but is related categorically to the word they are seeking. For example, one of my patients frequently asks for a pencil when filling out forms or jotting down notes to himself, though he really means a pen. Someone might say *bus* instead of *car*, or *pizza* instead of *hot dog*, or replace the word *rose* with *flower*. I have also often observed *anomia*, in which patients struggle to find the word they are looking for and feel it is on the tip of their tongue, or they recognize an object but give it the wrong name or are unable to name it. In a small percentage of cases, my long Covid patients have developed new stuttering disorders as well as halting and effortful speech. We're not sure why it occurs exactly but can see the way it can create problems beyond communication difficulties. Sometimes, people withdraw from conversations almost completely, embarrassed by their struggle to get words out, which may lead to social isolation, which, in turn, contributes to other maladies, such as depression.

Memory

Memory is arguably the most complex domain and refers to abilities across a spectrum that allow people to encode, store, and retrieve information. Components of memory include free recall (the retrieval of memories without any cues or prompting), cued recall (the retrieval of memories using aids such as cues, prompts, and reminders), recognition memory (the ability—in the present moment—to recognize that you've been previously exposed to a person, event, thing, or situation), semantic memory/autobiographical memory (facts about the world that have been gathered throughout our lives, such as what is the capital of Egypt, who was Canada's first prime minister, when was Shakespeare born, and memories of a personal nature, e.g., your first kiss, catching your first fish, watching the Pittsburgh Steelers play in the Super Bowl), long-term memory (storing information for a long period of time, whether it is conscious or explicit, or unconscious or implicit), and implicit learning (acquiring knowledge or the ability to learn something without intentionally trying to do so—such as learning to walk or to speak in one's native language, or knowing the words to a catchy Taylor Swift song).

Recently, I met with a patient who was battling with persistent memory problems approximately a year after contracting Covid. He loves the television show *Longmire,* a Western crime drama that follows a laconic sheriff as he rebuilds his life after the death of his wife. Filled with multiple storylines and plot twists, the show fascinates my patient, and yet he relayed to me that each new episode is a complete mystery to him as he cannot recall what happened even an episode or two before. He also has significant problems with misplacing his belongings and spends many hours a week hunting items down. Recently he bought an expensive pair of prescription sunglasses and, as he said, "set them down somewhere." He found them a few days later—in the refrigerator.

Perceptual-Motor Function

This domain refers to abilities required to both understand visual and spatial relationships among objects and to coordinate relevant motor skills. For example, someone may have a full range of movement in their arms, hands, and fingers, and yet find it impossible to button their shirt. They are unable to coordinate their visual perception of the buttons and buttonholes with the physical movements of their fingers. One of my patients planned and shopped for a cookout with friends and yet, when it came to putting together her brand-new grill, she just couldn't figure out the way the pieces fit together. After a couple of frustrating hours, she called a girlfriend for help. Prior to her Covid infection, this task would have taken her just a few minutes.

Perceptual-motor functioning declines significantly as people age, so observing decrements in elderly individuals can be expected, but seeing such issues in younger individuals may indicate a problem. In my clinic, when I hear my patients discussing such difficulties, I often ask them to draw a clock. This seemingly simple task involves many complex processes and can quickly help me see where a patient might need support. Struggles on a clock-drawing task are often a visual reminder of a patient's profound challenges and, in many cases, seeing their misdrawn clock can bring resistant patients around to the idea that they have significant cognitive concerns.

Social Cognition

This involves the processes used in the ways we perceive people in the world around us and how we interact with them. Dysfunction in this domain can manifest as socially inappropriate behavior such as a change in manners or expected behaviors during meals or in social settings. People might act in ways that are at odds with social norms, like standing up and shouting while at the movie theater. A change in personality or interests can occur, too. Perhaps a formerly outgoing person starts to withdraw from their social circle, or someone who once loved gardening seems happy to let weeds take over their pristine flowerbeds. Sometimes people can become overly trusting of strangers, lacking the social awareness and perception they once had. In recent years, I've had numerous patients fall prey to scams of various kinds, as they are often unable to differentiate between what is true and what is obviously false. My elderly father received a phone call from someone claiming to be his grandchild who told him he was in another state, was involved in a car accident, and needed $1,000 wired to him urgently. Luckily, my father checked in with me and didn't fall for the scam but to an individual with cognitive impairment who has difficulties evaluating nuance and social context, the situation may have seemed plausible, and the story might have ended differently.

COGNITIVE IMPAIRMENT IN DAILY LIFE

Cognitive difficulties due to long Covid can occur in one domain or several, making it challenging to get through the day as they invariably show up in what are called instrumental activities of daily living (IADLs). More complex than basic activities of daily living (e.g., eating, bathing, toileting), IADLs contribute to a person's quality of life, both at home and beyond, in the wider community, and the impact of cognitive dysfunction can be severe. IADLs can include care of others, care of pets, being able to communicate with others via phone or email, driving and transportation, health management, hobbies, looking after a home, meal preparation and cleanup, personal finance, religious and spiritual activities, and shopping.

In cases where people are extremely cognitively impaired, functional problems are easy to see — reflected in such behaviors as putting pants on backward, forgetting how to use a car key, trying to microwave food in the washing machine, or displaying striking personality changes often marked by patterns of suspicion and paranoia. In cases of milder forms of cognitive impairment, daily functioning is influenced in more subtle and nuanced ways, including forgetting details of conversations, misplacing items, and having difficulty sustaining focus. Sometimes long haulers (or their family members) may be reluctant to acknowledge that their struggles might be attributed to cognitive dysfunction caused by long Covid, or they may be unsure how to recognize their symptoms as signs that they need help. They may think their cognitive "slips" are due to fatigue, stress, distraction, or being overwhelmed, or might consider them a natural part of the aging process. However, there are various behavioral red flags that are suggestive of abnormal cognitive function, and I provide information here to help you observe and track these possible signs.

Looking for Red Flags

These common daily activities can be impeded or influenced by cognitive impairment in various ways, and it can be a good idea to keep an eye on — and a record of — any recent changes in behavior you may have noticed:

- Driving: Problems include forgetting to check mirrors before setting out or during driving, displaying poor speed control (driving well below the speed limit or frequently speeding up and slowing down), making a left turn without looking, failing to stay in a lane, or failing to verify a blind spot. In addition, people may often lose track of where they parked their car, lose their car keys, or struggle with the steps for filling up the car with gas.

- Finances: There may be issues with bill paying, including failing to pay bills on time or at all, or paying the same bill multiple times. Credit cards and bank cards may be misplaced as may important financial documents such as receipts, car titles, insurance information, etc. People may be more likely to fall prey to investment fraud or other financial scams.

- Healthcare: Issues may include a lack of knowledge about health conditions or an inability to effectively use medical devices (e.g., asthma inhalers, CPAP masks), read and comprehend prescription drug labels, or follow directions for dosage. Appointments may be missed and follow-up visits unscheduled and there may be an inability to provide a linear or coherent medical history.

- Social functioning: There may be a misinterpretation of social cues, disregard for social norms in conversation (interrupting others, invading others' personal space when talking, etc.), difficulty in staying focused in conversations, and veering off on tangentially related topics. Some people may become increasingly socially withdrawn.

- Cooking/grocery shopping: These activities may appear simple and yet are cognitively complex, involving many processes and steps. Issues may show up in more obvious examples, such as forgetting to turn off the stove, or they may be more nuanced: frequently burning meals, restarting preparation of the same dish multiple times due to difficulty following a recipe, leaving a plastic spatula on a hot plate, or finding it challenging to plan and execute a complex holiday dinner, particularly if this hasn't previously been an issue. When shopping, signs of cognitive impairment may include taking a very long time to pick up just a few items at the store, forgetting the layout of a familiar store, perseverating (getting cognitively "stuck") on what to purchase, using a self-checkout and leaving with your groceries without paying, or losing receipts.

- Technology: Be aware of frequent difficulties with remembering computer passwords and getting locked out of accounts, repeated spelling errors in emails or online posts, reposting the same information, or an inability to recognize real news accounts from parodies. People may also constantly lose their phones or TV remotes and may find them stored in unusual places such as the bread box or bathroom cabinet.

NEXT STEPS

When long Covid survivors demonstrate red flags that could be indicative of cognitive impairment, it is time to consider an evaluation. In general, if new behaviors, noted consistently over a period of a few weeks, cause you to wonder about cognitive decline in yourself or a family member, it is best to reach out to a primary care provider for an initial appointment (or to make an appointment with a post-Covid clinic). You may find it helpful at this point to reread Chapter 1 to prepare for a visit. It will be especially important to keep track of symptoms and behaviors that have led you to suspect cognitive dysfunction.

Cognitive Testing

At your visit with your doctor, you can expect (or ask for) a brief cognitive assessment. This is typically carried out using one of the following screening tools:

- Mini-Mental State Examination (MMSE): This test is made up of simple questions and problems, including the time and place of the test, repetition of word lists, math such as counting down from one hundred in sevens (serial sevens), language use and comprehension, and basic motor skills.

- Montreal Cognitive Assessment (MoCA): This is a short assessment with eleven sections that test a patient's ability with language, verbal fluency, visuospatial tasks, memory, attention, recall, abstract thinking, and orientation to time and place.
- Clock-Drawing Test: As mentioned, this quick assessment tool tests for several domains of cognition, including perceptual-motor function, attention, and executive functioning. Typically, the patient is given instructions such as, "Please draw a clock, putting in all the numbers on the clock and showing the time twenty after ten."
- Informant Questionnaire on Cognitive Decline in the Elderly (IQCODE): This quick assessment is done with an "informant"— usually a family member or caregiver who knows a patient well— and is given at an appointment with the patient present. Designed to be used with adults of all ages (despite its name), it simply asks a respondent to rate how much an individual has declined in key areas of cognitive and daily functioning over a fixed period. The IQCODE is often combined with other screening measures to provide a fuller picture of a patient's cognitive status.

These tests often identify the presence of moderate or severe cognitive problems and, if these are observed, your doctor would refer you to a specialist (I discuss this in full on the pages that follow). However, the standard tests may not be sufficiently sensitive to identify mild difficulties, especially when used with previously high-functioning people. They should be interpreted thoughtfully and with caution by your doctor as one step toward reaching a diagnosis and should not be used, especially in the absence of other information, to conclude that someone with cognitive complaints and/or functional problems is fully cognitively normal. If you feel that your doctor does not understand or accept your concerns, it's important that you let them know and ask for a referral to a specialist, such as a neuropsychologist or a neurologist for a more comprehensive evaluation.

While referrals to specialists are often important, not everyone needs them and sometimes they can be triggered too quickly, creating unnecessary anxiety, and exhausting limited resources. More than a decade ago, I was involved in a landmark research study at the CIBS Center known as the ABC Trial, a practice-changing investigation that demonstrated that interrupting sedation in critically ill patients on ventilators led to better outcomes, as continuous sedation could contribute to cognitive dysfunction (and other problems).[24] One of my roles was to carry out neuropsychological testing on every patient at hospital discharge and I found that 100 percent of these individuals had cognitive impairment according to psychometric testing. However, in the three months that followed, about two in three of them made significant progress as their acute health concerns improved and further cognitive testing showed they were within the range of normal. I learned an important lesson during this experience. Ignoring cognitive problems is a concern, but labeling symptoms as an issue too quickly, especially solely on the basis of cognitive testing, is also unwise.

In my practice, if patients display mild abnormalities on cognitive screening tests but indicate that their functioning is intact, I tend to adopt a "watchful waiting" approach, as many mild problems naturally resolve. I schedule a follow-up appointment for three to six months later to reevaluate the situation while letting the patient know they can contact me before then if they notice any changes. If, on the other hand, a patient earns scores reflecting clear abnormalities (as did a patient of mine who earned a score of 18 out of 30 on the MoCA after a stay in the Covid ICU) or reports substantial functional changes typically persisting for three to six months, then, regardless of their score, I usually refer them for a more comprehensive evaluation.

SEEING A SPECIALIST

Your doctor may refer you to a particular specialist or may recommend a specific practice or hospital, leaving you to find one that seems a good fit for you. Specialists can be found in many medium-sized and large cities, throughout most healthcare systems, and they typically accept different kinds of health insurance.

Neuropsychologist

Neuropsychologists (like me) are licensed psychologists or researchers who have received specialized training that enables them to understand the relationship between the brain and behavior, to determine an individual's cognitive status, and to characterize the nature and severity of cognitive impairment, if it is present. Like our clinical psychology colleagues, we are skilled at conducting diagnostic interviews and history-taking but much of our work involves the use and interpretation of detailed and comprehensive neuropsychological tests. These range from relatively abbreviated but still challenging test batteries, such as the forty-five-minute Repeatable Battery for the Assessment of Neuropsychological Status, to very lengthy evaluations that can take a full day or even more. Sometimes a patient may undergo testing over several days, as the process can be physically taxing and emotionally exhausting.

Unlike the brief screening tools referred to earlier, the tests that comprise a neuropsychological evaluation are highly sensitive in detecting even mild cognitive deficits and in discriminating between normal and abnormal forms of cognition. They are designed to evaluate a wide array of domains or, in some cases, to evaluate in detail specific domains such as memory or attention. Usually, these tests are done using paper and pencil but increasingly they are carried out on computers or iPads. Sometimes, neuropsychological tests are augmented by tests assessing mental health conditions including anxiety, depression, and PTSD and, in some cases, by personality tests. Using data obtained from these tests combined with information derived from conversations with patients and their families or caregivers, neuropsychologists can determine where cognitive problems exist, explain the implications of such problems, and offer guidance about treatments and other relevant next steps.

It is important to highlight here the need to have evaluations that assess a full array of abilities and not just one or two. Anything less than this is more of a cognitive screening than a truly comprehensive examination. As I often counsel patients, it is perfectly appropriate to ask to speak to a neuropsychologist prior to your testing to understand what you are about to embark on—which areas of functioning will be evaluated, how long the testing will take, how thorough it will be, what kind of feedback you will receive, etc. While examinations can take many different forms, it is important that they are designed to answer the questions that you and/or your primary care physician (PCP) have.

Neurologist

Neurologists, unlike neuropsychologists, are physicians, and have received training in internal medicine and advanced training in the medical dimensions of brain dysfunction and disease. They are a diverse group of professionals and often specialize in treating particular conditions such as epilepsy, movement disorders, and neuro-oncology. If pursuing a long Covid evaluation from a neurologist, cognitive or behavioral neurologists are best equipped to evaluate cognitive complaints after Covid-19 as their focus is cognitive and behavioral challenges stemming from a neurologic condition.

In seeking a diagnosis, neurologists usually send for bloodwork to rule out reversible forms of cognitive decline (e.g., hypothyroidism, electrolyte imbalances, B_{12} deficiency, medications), arrange for brain imaging to look for structural deficits, an EEG (if appropriate) to rule out occult seizures, and neuropsychological testing to evaluate the pattern of memory and cognitive deficit. Sometimes they will assess a patient's mood and/or sleep and consider if and how these need to be treated. In some cases, such as instances in which patients have had rapid and precipitous cognitive decline—as has been observed in rare cases in long haulers—neurologists may perform workups for specific potential causes, evaluating conditions such as normal-pressure hydrocephalus, viral encephalitis, and prion disease.

Sometimes patients may be referred to both neuropsychology and neurology as experts in these fields have complementary skills that, when combined, lead to the best clinical insights, the most accurate diagnoses, and the most optimal patient care. I generally encourage other professionals to refer to both specialists if they can, while acknowledging at times that it may be more than a patient needs. In some cases, specific clinical questions dictate referrals to one specialist or another.

Speech and Language Pathologist

Speech and language pathologists (SLPs) are typically master's level professionals who work with patients experiencing difficulties with speech and language, and cognitive issues more broadly. They are often viewed as experts in the treatment of communication problems such as aphasia or stuttering but their training, often grounded in neuroscience and the assessment of cognition, makes them well equipped to provide a wide range of services—primarily cognitive rehabilitation therapy—to people with cognitive impairment of all kinds. For this reason, many long Covid survivors are referred to SLPs after reporting cognitive complaints or if an initial screening test has suggested cognitive abnormalities.

SLPs may perform brief cognitive assessments of patients to help inform treatment plans, and although these are usually longer than a simple MMSE or a MoCA, they are less comprehensive than the evaluations done by a neuropsychologist. SLPs will often refer their patients for neuropsychological evaluations if they need to further understand the complexities and nuances of a patient's condition.

In many cases, SLPs work in hospital-based clinics, either in the department of rehabilitation medicine (also known as the department of physical medicine and rehabilitation) or the department of neurology, and, in some instances, they work in specialized inpatient rehabilitation hospitals where they see outpatients, often via telemedicine. Presently, few SLPs are integrated into long Covid clinics, and I hope this can change in the future. Their services are usually covered by insurance, although objective evidence of cognitive impairment, even if done using very rudimentary testing, is required. In my experience, SLPs who have worked with brain-injured and post-concussive patients are particularly enthusiastic about seeing Covid long haulers, believing— as I do—that they have many tools at their disposal to treat and improve their cognitive impairment.

Occupational Therapist

Like SLPs, occupational therapists (OTs) are generally master's trained professionals who are experts in helping patients find ways to adapt to new challenges due to chronic illness or injury by learning new skills or recovering old ones. Occupational therapists work in many different environments, often in general hospital or specialty hospital clinics, and they have unique expertise in "functional cognitive assessment," which focuses on determining how cognitive impairment impedes a patient's ability to engage in daily activities. Frequently, their approaches extend beyond the clinic into the real world. While training in cognitive rehabilitation, I observed a typical assessment in which the OT escorted a patient to the grocery store, gave them a complicated shopping list and a budget, and observed them from a distance, noting how efficiently they followed directions or whether they were able to make sense of them at all. This approach provides valuable insights into both a patient's abilities and deficits in ways that are difficult to capture in a typical neuropsychological evaluation. An OT's assessment often works hand in hand with those performed by a neuropsychologist. Many long Covid patients have found the involvement of an occupational therapist invaluable in their care and recovery.

A SAMPLE APPOINTMENT

When my patient Megan arrived for her appointment, she had already done neuropsychological testing and received a diagnosis of mild cognitive impairment. While this is a correct diagnosis, it can seem misleading because, as my patients have often noted, there is nothing "mild" about it. I was pleased that Megan's testing covered the six key domains described in this chapter, using carefully selected tests known to be reliable, valid, and sensitive in identifying deficits. A patient is likely to have much better results if we can see exactly where their cognitive struggles are showing up in testing. In some cases, I see patients who have not undergone comprehensive testing and I refer them to receive it, and in others, as with Megan, the testing has already been done.

My aim with Megan, and many patients like her, was to support her while she was undergoing significant changes, to guide her understanding of these challenges while considering the data from her cognitive evaluation, to find a way to treat her cognitive dysfunction, and to help her cope with the mental health difficulties resulting from the many upheavals in her life. I find that trying to understand a patient's challenges in isolation is almost always a mistake and with long Covid patients, cognitive issues and mental health problems often coexist. For the sake of simplicity, I address them in different chapters in the book, but it is important to remember that they are often intertwined, each impacted by the other to varying degrees.

In Megan's first session, we aimed to devise a plan, shaped and informed, as it should be whenever possible, by data from her cognitive testing. In her case, she had wide-ranging strengths and weaknesses, displaying the "scattershot" pattern so typical among people with illness-related cognitive impairment. This pattern usually displays abilities that are at or above expected levels as well as general deficits that range from mild to severe, reflecting problems in multiple brain regions as opposed to just one. Megan showed significant deficits in nearly all aspects of the attention domain, including impairment in her ability to sustain her focus for long periods of time and to shift quickly from one task to another. She also had processing speed deficits and impaired executive functioning, while her memory appeared to be largely intact. The testing confirmed what she was experiencing in her life with her inability to complete her master's thesis and her difficulties at work. Yes, she had memory problems in her day-to-day life, but it appeared that they probably resulted from deficits in attention and slow processing speed rather than from fundamental inabilities in memory.

By the end of Megan's first session, I was able to begin to understand her story and her needs, and to develop a treatment plan—one that continues to unfold as we assess and reassess her progress. There was a sense of relief in her eyes as we talked about next steps. "I'm so glad I did the testing," she said. "Though it was scary." I nodded, acknowledging the courageous step she had made in seeking help for the difficulties she was experiencing. Now, after seeing her primary care physician, getting a referral, and undergoing a battery of tests, she was in a position to move forward with personalized treatment based on the findings.

My hope is that if you or someone you know has cognitive symptoms, you are now in a position to find help. Once an evaluation and testing have taken place, you will have insight into the scope and extent of deficits, and a path forward toward recovery. In the next chapter, I discuss different options for cognitive rehabilitation and show the ways that cognitive difficulties can be effectively addressed.

CHAPTER 3

REHABILITATING AND RESTORING:
Improving Cognitive Functioning in Long Haulers

One day in early 2022, in the throes of the pandemic, I logged on to Twitter and noticed a message in my inbox. Sent by a speech and language pathologist in Auburn, Alabama, the words echoed those of so many of us in healthcare: that the cognitive dysfunction she was observing daily in Covid-19 survivors was a "much bigger problem than anyone seems to realize." That resonated deeply with me, but it was her next sentence that really struck a chord. She was greatly troubled that many of the cognitive issues she was seeing could be readily improved—and yet there was little mention anywhere of available treatments. I found myself agreeing, and, since then, have continued this conversation with her and many other medical professionals from various disciplines.

The popular and quite discouraging narrative that there are "no treatments for long Covid" emerged during the early part of the pandemic and has persisted. This statement has been repeated so frequently and circulated so widely that it is often accepted as the absolute truth, to the great detriment of many people. Perhaps you have heard these words yourself and have become disheartened. While it's accurate to say that many features of long Covid remain mysterious and intractable and, in multiple areas, doctors are still navigating their way through new terrain, leaving many people without relief for debilitating symptoms, when it comes to cognitive deficits in domains such as attention, executive functioning, and memory, there are already evidence-based methods and strategies in place that can help patients get better. Over the past couple of years, I have treated a vast number of long Covid patients struggling with cognitive impairment and, over time, I have seen their functioning improve. In this chapter, I look at different options for cognitive rehabilitation and put you in a position to advocate for treatment for yourself or someone you know.

In the late 1990s, pioneering neuroscientist Dr. Ramona Hopkins documented the severe cognitive impairment experienced by patients who had survived acute respiratory distress syndrome.[1] Later, my colleagues and I found that during ICU stays, one in three survivors of critical illness developed cognitive problems as severe as those seen in people with traumatic brain injuries or mild dementia.[2] Yet when Dr. Hopkins and I asked our hundreds of patients whether they had ever been referred for cognitive rehabilitation, the answer was a universally resounding *no*.

At the time, my clinical research led me to ask questions sitting at kitchen tables, in living rooms, and on covered front porches in the urban centers and, more often, hills and hollows of rural Alabama, Georgia, Kentucky, and Tennessee. As I crisscrossed the mid-south, armed with a clipboard, a stopwatch, and a few #2 pencils, I learned the ways that cognitive impairment impacted people's lives after critical illness through narratives of jobs lost, disability claims denied, and vital relationships fractured. The people telling me these stories, sometimes through tears, were research subjects in clinical investigations into post-intensive care syndrome — and they had become my friends, their names, faces, and hopes for the future transcending the study numbers they were given. I could not believe so little was being done to help improve their neuropsychological functioning.

There were surely complex reasons for this, grounded, at least in part, in a limited appreciation among physicians of the extent to which medical illness can cause cognitive impairment and in popular understandings of brain injuries that we now know are very narrow. A soldier in a war zone standing too close to a blast explosion, a football player knocked unconscious by a helmet-to-helmet hit, a house painter falling off a ladder and fracturing their skull: these were all easily identified as scenarios that might cause brain injuries and would surely have resulted in appointments with specialists and follow-up care. In contrast, illness-induced cognitive changes were met with a collective shrug.

In the last twenty years or so, a shift has occurred in understanding the scope of brain injuries and the integration of cognitive rehabilitation into the care of patients with illnesses of many kinds. A recent PubMed search into research studies on cognitive rehabilitation revealed that in 2021, twenty-three were published on cancer, thirty-two on multiple sclerosis, and 259 on cognitive rehabilitation in general, a 1,000 percent increase over the twenty-three studies published in 2000. This should mean that more and more patients with cognitive deficits, including those with long Covid, are now able to engage in effective treatments aimed at improving their neuropsychological challenges, and yet these treatments are far too often failing to reach people that need them. Just recently, I was contacted by a marketing executive from Canada and a therapist from New York City who were looking for treatment for, as they put it, their "brain fog." They were both thoughtful and motivated people with access to healthcare and resources who were completely unaware that cognitive rehabilitation existed and that it could potentially improve their brain functioning. Their experience is repeated countless times across the country—and around the world.

It's true that little formal research has been published on the effects of cognitive rehabilitation on survivors of Covid-19 but it is a huge and consequential mistake to conclude that this means it will not work. As

I said in Chapter 2, we've known for decades that some medical conditions, including viral infections, contribute to cognitive problems, and we've also known that the kind of cognitive dysfunction that develops in response to acute and chronic illness—deficits in areas such as attention, executive functioning, and processing speed—is responsive to cognitive rehabilitation. While Covid-19 has its own "fingerprint," most experts would agree that *cognitive problems are cognitive problems* and that it is likely that cognitive rehabilitation, so helpful to people with other conditions, will be effective for those with long Covid, too. Although my clinical research rarely takes place around kitchen tables these days, I continue to see the impact of cognitive impairment in the lives of many people, especially those living with long Covid. Now I, and many others, have the means to help.

In the previous chapter, I discussed different kinds of cognitive dysfunction and how they may appear in daily life, how to seek an initial evaluation from a specialist, and what to expect at your appointment. Here, I'll lay out possible cognitive rehabilitation treatment therapies that are available to help to address cognitive impairment and that I find extremely effective with my patients.

While cognitive rehabilitation can be very helpful, it's important to note that long Covid patients who meet the criteria for ME/CFS can easily become extremely fatigued and experience post-exertional malaise (PEM). Exercise, including cognitive exercise or brain exertion, can cause them harm. Be aware that pushing through feelings of mental fatigue can be detrimental to your recovery so listen to your body and rest as needed. Some people use apps such as Visible (makevisible .com) to track their symptoms, exertion, and to pace their activity, but if fatigue is a key symptom for you, it is best to check in with your doctor before starting cognitive rehabilitation.

In general, cognitive rehabilitation is guided by two fundamental principles: 1) that individuals have the ability to modify and adjust behavior after experiencing changes to their brain, and 2) that one of the brain's key features is plasticity, which allows it to recover following damage. These principles inform two general approaches to treatment—compensatory and restorative—that are implemented in wide-ranging ways through various paradigms, techniques, and methods.

Compensatory approaches use behavioral tools or environmental modifications to reduce, limit, or avoid the impact of cognitive deficits, in order to help people function more effectively and independently. Strategies can be internal (using rhymes to aid memory, learning to break down complex tasks into smaller pieces) or external (diaries, notebooks, lists, planners, and even virtual assistants such as Alexa, Siri, or Google). Restorative approaches, in contrast, aim to recover an individual's cognitive capacities by harnessing the brain's ability to modify its structure and function and to build new connections. Increasingly, restorative strategies involve brain training through specialized games played on personal electronic devices. While these compensatory and restorative approaches are distinct, they can certainly be complementary and are often used together in the treatment of patients.

In some cases, after careful consideration, healthcare professionals may prescribe medication, such as a low-dose stimulant, to help with attention deficits. However, it is best used to supplement cognitive rehabilitation therapies, not to replace them.

COMPENSATORY REHABILITATION

Tasha is one of the many patients I've been fortunate to get to know since the start of the pandemic, having met her at a conference where she was advocating for long Covid patients like herself. A young professional managing a team of employees in a small startup and an active soccer mom, she liked to relax by making complicated meals for her family. Recently, however, she had started to find it hard to follow recipes, often missing steps or ingredients, with haphazard results, and at work her inbox overflowed with unanswered emails and unfinished projects. She had contracted Covid at a birthday party and although her physical functioning had rebounded after the acute phase of her illness, cognitive problems were lingering. She decided a visit to her general practitioner would be a good idea and, thankfully, her doctor really listened to her concerns and referred her to a behavioral neurologist who conducted neuropsychological testing. During a diagnostic evaluation, Tasha struggled, demonstrating problems across a range of cognitive domains. Like so many long Covid patients, she was diagnosed with mild cognitive impairment.

Far too often, the story ends there but this thoughtful provider referred Tasha to a multi-specialty rehabilitation hospital for outpatient cognitive rehabilitation. Now, several months later, Tasha is starting to see improvements. In conversations with coworkers and anyone who wants to listen, she talks about strategies she has learned to rely on—such as using sticky notes for reminders and avoiding pressure-packed situations that increase the odds of her making mistakes. Her supervisor joked with her the other day, observing that Tasha was "even more organized" now than before and, although this was not strictly true, it felt good to have someone note how well she had integrated insights from rehabilitation into her daily life.

Tasha learned her new skills during five months of twice-weekly outpatient sessions of cognitive rehabilitation with a focus on compensatory techniques. First used, in a more rudimentary form, during World War I with soldiers experiencing traumatic brain injuries, compensatory cognitive rehabilitation has been shown to be effective in many clinical populations experiencing cognitive deficits due to conditions such as cancer,[3] multiple sclerosis,[4] Parkinson's disease, fibromyalgia, mild traumatic brain injuries,[5] post-intensive care syndrome,[6] and stroke, and I've seen it work especially well with survivors of critical illness struggling with cognitive impairment. Compensatory therapies, typically delivered by speech and language pathologists or occupational therapists, focus on creating individualized tools and strategies that can be integrated into a patient's daily life to help with specific struggles and compensate for deficits, particularly in areas such as attention, executive functioning, and aspects of memory.

A key element of this approach is the understanding and use of metacognitive strategies. Simply stated, these help people to "think about thinking," to develop an awareness of their thought processes, including strengths and weaknesses, and to learn to actively adapt their thinking. For example, being aware of a tendency to forget people's names or that you take longer than anticipated to get out of the house for a doctor's appointment can pave the way for solutions. With repetition and practice, the mechanisms become second nature, helping to reduce the impact of impairment, and to maximize existing strengths to improve functioning at home, school, work, and other areas of life valued by patients.

During Tasha's personalized cognitive rehabilitation program, she worked harder than she thought she could, pushed hard and lovingly supported by a team that included an occupational therapist and a speech and language pathologist, working in tandem to help improve her functioning. In her testing, Tasha's most severe difficulties had showed up in the cognitive domains of attention, executive functioning, and memory, and her team worked to improve these areas. Initially, she was skeptical of the value of suggested tools such as planners, reluctant to believe that they could be of any use, and yet she took them on board, using bright color-coded tabs in a binder that she studiously kept in one place. Sticky notes became a saving grace, messages scrawled on strategically arranged squares of paper, including one that she noticed each time she sat in her chair and leaned her head back in exasperation. It read "Do One Thing at a Time."

Another especially helpful tool was a technique that taught her to take a moment to think when she was spending too much time on a task or was about to be sidetracked from a goal. During a recent baking session, she had struggled for an hour with a favorite chocolate fudge cake recipe and was starting over for the third time when she paused and said "Stop!" to herself. After a moment, she was able to see that she was being distracted by the TV news, her kids playing in another room, and the distant sound of her neighbor mowing her lawn. There was too much going on to focus on the cake. She sighed. She would need to wait for a quieter time to bake—but now was a perfect moment to see what the kids were up to.

Metacognitive Strategies

Many of the metacognitive strategies used with great success by Tasha and other long Covid patients whom my colleagues and I work with are found in Goal Management Training (GMT), an evidence-based, in-person approach to cognitive rehabilitation that I'm particularly passionate about. A widely investigated behavioral treatment for deficits in areas such as executive functioning, GMT was developed at the UK Medical Research Council at Cambridge University in the mid-1990s by neuropsychologist Dr. Ian Robertson[7] and modified into its current form by my friend and research colleague Dr. Brian Levine, and Dr. Tom Manly.[8] I learned a great deal about this approach to therapy while studying cognitive rehabilitation at the Oliver Zangwill Center in England more than a decade ago, and while thinking about it conjures up memories of cobblestone streets lined with fish and chip shops and high teas with lively colleagues in leafy gardens, there are more objective reasons to endorse it. Robust evidence supports its effectiveness among varied patient demographics and, for this reason, while there are other strategic and metacognitive approaches that could be discussed, I'll focus my comments on GMT.

Taught to patients in either individual or group settings, GMT provides a systematic approach to carrying out everyday tasks by helping people understand the specific way their mind works and how to recognize situations when difficulties may arise for them, and offers effective coping methods. Armed with new insights into their own thought processes and with a menu of internal strategies to choose from, they can reduce making frustrating mistakes and improve planning, memory, and focus.

Many aspects of GMT have been particularly helpful to my patients over the years, and I've seen my long Covid patients incorporate them into their lives and find them extremely useful. The following three techniques are especially valuable.

Present-Mindedness

Many of the cognitive mistakes people make occur because they are not giving their full attention to whatever they are currently doing. Known as "absentminded errors," they often happen when someone is not operating in the present moment—their mind is elsewhere. Perhaps they are thinking about a recent conversation—as I was one day when I drove away from a gas station with the nozzle still in my car, pulling the hose off the gas pump—or about an upcoming work meeting. Whatever it is, it means they are inattentive to their immediate surroundings. These slipups often occur at predictable times, such as when we are rushing around, feeling stressed, or fatigued. While everyone experiences slipups, people with cognitive dysfunction experience them far more regularly, which proves disruptive to their lives. Learning "present-mindedness" as a way of reducing slipups can become a valuable tool. It begins with recognizing the situations in which slipups occur and being aware that you may be vulnerable to them in similar future scenarios. By noticing when your thoughts are starting to wander, it is possible to self-correct and focus on the present.

One of my patients, Malik, a middle-aged unemployed healthcare worker recently diagnosed with long Covid, had seen several specialists at the medical center before heading home. He lived several hours from Nashville and wanted to arrive before dark. More than two hours into his journey, he suddenly realized that he had forgotten to stop by the hospital pharmacy to pick up his newly prescribed medications. Now, sitting in a truck stop as dusk crept in, he lay his head on the steering wheel and wept. The pharmacy was already closed, and he would have to make the three-hundred-mile round trip to Nashville all over again the next day—or find a way to transfer the prescriptions to his local but out-of-state pharmacy. Either way, it was a disaster. In his mind, he could see himself hurrying from the clinic toward the parking garage, thinking over his appointments, his distressing financial situation, and the fact that his truck needed fuel. He had walked right past the pharmacy on his way to the car. Overwhelmed by worry, exhausted, and in a rush, he was primed to be forgetful and inattentive.

In our work together, Malik has started to understand that there are situations in which he is especially likely to make such absentminded slipups, and, with increased self-awareness, he is learning to anticipate them and to operate in a present-minded way, with a heightened sense of focus on the moment at hand and by allowing fewer distractions.

Splitting Tasks into Subtasks

People who develop executive dysfunction have significant difficulties with planning and initiating, and when they encounter cognitively challenging tasks, they often don't know where to start. They may respond by doing nothing or, in contrast, they may "jump in," feeling that they have to act, but their approach may not address the issue in helpful or logical ways. These patterns frequently plague people with long Covid who often find themselves overwhelmed by daily tasks, especially if there are many component parts to contend with, such as preparing a holiday meal for a group, applying for a job, signing up for classes, planning a trip, or setting up a bank account. One key to successful functioning and task completion is learning to divide tasks into small and cognitively manageable subtasks.

My patient Savannah was reduced to panic and paralysis any time she faced a project with many moving parts. "I just couldn't see my way through," she'd say, and often that would lead to her avoiding any aspect of the task. It was just insurmountable for her. When her attorney was helping with her disability application, there were so many documents to read and forms to fill out that Savannah had no idea where to start and often showed up to consultations stressed and unprepared. Over time and with much practice, Savannah learned—as I liked to say to her—to "eat an elephant one bite at a time" by breaking large and seemingly overwhelming tasks into small, achievable ones.

Checking (Stop and Think)

On my fortieth birthday, far longer ago than I would like, my wife, Michelle, bought me a watch with the word *Relax* written across the stainless-steel wristband. At the time, I was in the early days of my research career, helping to raise three young children, teaching a Sunday School class or two, and generally struggling to keep my head above water as I was pulled in countless directions. As I went about my day, I noticed the simple message ("Relax") dozens of times—when I turned the key to start my car, or did pull-ups at the gym, or picked up a bag of groceries—and each time, I'd pause to breathe, reflect, and, sometimes, reorient.

I'm reminded of this story when I think of "Checking (stop and think)," a life-changing strategy for many patients who use it to pause and reflect on what they are doing and whether it will help them achieve their desired goal. With time and practice, they can check in with themselves, to stop and think and adjust, as necessary, to be more effective—just as Tasha did when making her chocolate cake, realizing that trying again later in the day might more likely lead to baking success. In Malik's case, before heading home after his medical appointments, he has learned to make a deliberate effort to stop and reflect on whether there is anything he needs to attend to before leaving the campus. Encouraged by positive results with this approach, he has started using it almost everywhere—at the doctor's office, where he paused and thought about whether he had any more questions; at the grocery store, where he reflected on whether he had picked up everything on his list; and before leaving home, checking that he has his wallet, keys, and medication, as necessary.

External Aids

While GMT and similar programs teach strategies that patients can internalize and take on board to modify their thinking and behavior, another important compensatory tool, and one that has also played a key part in Tasha's story, is the use of external aids. These are resources, sometimes technological, that a patient can use or engage with to work around some of their cognitive challenges. It's true that patients and their families sometimes roll their eyes at the idea that external aids could be helpful, especially when someone's life circumstances may have dramatically changed because of cognitive impairment but, at their best, when used frequently and with intention, they can be transformative, especially when adapted and tailored to a patient's particular needs. They can bring structure into the lives of cognitively impaired patients that enable them to function more effectively by helping to offset deficits. Examples of external aids that SLPs often introduce are:

- Post–it Notes
- Checklists, which may include shopping lists, lists of medications, appointments, and steps to take when engaging in a routine
- Calendars (one of my research patients has calendars covering almost every wall of her house—perhaps not the most efficient strategy but it works very well for her)
- Whiteboards
- Notebooks
- Medication containers that contain daily pill selections
- Smartphones and/or smartwatches—with alarms set as reminders, calendars, timers, etc.
- Intelligent virtual assistants such as Alexa and Google Home

While evidence strongly supports the benefits of external aids, they work best if used deliberately and consistently. Often rehabilitation specialists will help develop comprehensive strategies for their patients for the use of these aids, taking into account their specific deficits, and will provide training in how to use them, follow up on how they are working, and modifying treatment plans as needed. Often lists, notebooks, calendars, etc., are stored in a prominent place in an individual's home or workplace and are used at specific times every day. The aids can take some time to get used to, and patients may need motivation to get started and keep going with them before they see changes. A specialist can be an excellent support in both the practical and emotional side of rehabilitation.

Treatment Length

In many cases, both metacognitive strategies and external aids are used to help a patient, but interventions will vary depending on the nature of deficits. The time it takes to make progress differs from patient to patient, but an SLP who works extensively with long haulers advised me that a standard treatment protocol is ten to twelve weekly one-hour sessions, though some patients are seen for six to twelve months.

RESTORATIVE REHABILITATION

Restorative training offers a very different and, in many ways, complementary method of improving brain functioning. Instead of compensating for a person's cognitive deficits by using internal and external strategies and tools, it aims to restore or strengthen the brain's performance, thus enhancing cognitive function. A once controversial approach with growing scientific support, it is grounded in contemporary understandings of neuroplasticity—the brain's ability to grow, evolve, and, crucially, repair itself after injuries and insults of various kinds—and widely popularized by neuropsychiatrist Dr. Norman Doidge in his classic book *The Brain That Changes Itself.*

The brain's capacity to rewire itself lies at the heart of restorative approaches to cognitive rehabilitation for those with acquired brain injuries and other forms of cognitive impairment, including people with illness-induced cognitive impairment. Advocates believe, based on scientific evidence, that when someone's brain is challenged in focused, demanding, and sustained ways through engagement with specially designed video games and computerized programs known as brain games, growth and change occurs, new neuronal connections are made, and cognition strengthens in much the same way as muscles do after physical exercise.

Skeptics still question the value of this approach, and some important points need clarifying regarding the durability of improvements, whether they sustain over time and after treatment is stopped, and if they transfer to other tasks. But the evidence supporting the benefits is too compelling to dismiss out of hand. In addition, this treatment can take place in a patient's home and doesn't require a therapist appointment, making it potentially available to huge numbers of people, including those who may find it difficult to access conventional therapy. This is an especially important consideration as specialists like SLPs and occupational therapists are a scarce resource around the world. If safe, effective, and affordable innovative models of treatment exist, we should embrace them.

Neuroplasticity-Based Restorative Training in Action

In the early days of the pandemic, we at Vanderbilt Medical Center, along with colleagues at Weill Cornell Medical Center and NewYork-Presbyterian Hospital, partnered with Akili Interactive, a technology company, to design studies on whether neuroplasticity-based restorative rehabilitation could be used to treat cognitive problems in Covid long haulers.[9] While compensatory approaches have been studied for much of a century, there are very few studies that explore the impact of restorative rehabilitation. At Vanderbilt, my team launched the CONTACT Trial, a small, randomized, controlled clinical trial that, as a "feasibility study," will help us figure out whether bigger studies can be effectively carried out in the future. Participants play EndeavorRx, a specially designed video game that targets the cognitive domain of attention with a specific focus on processing speed. Originally created to help children with attention-deficit/hyperactivity disorder (ADHD), it is now FDA-approved as an ADHD treatment for children ages eight to twelve.[10] We hope to find out if it will be similarly effective in treating cognitive impairment in long haulers.

Ayumi's Story

Ayumi, a technology executive in her early thirties, struggled with cognitive difficulties after contracting Covid. She found herself in the hospital for a few days in early 2021 and though she bounced back physically and returned to work, she noticed cognitive problems about a month after discharge. Complicated reports, rich with dense information about market trends and predictions, used to be easy bedtime reading for her but now, working her way through one reminded her of the day she hiked the first leg of the 2,650-mile Pacific Crest Trail—it was exhausting and seemed to go on forever. Thinking on her feet had become challenging, too. In meetings where she could once command the room and consistently impress with the depth of her knowledge, she struggled to find the data or the words she was seeking.

The day she learned she was eligible for the CONTACT Trial, she sobbed into her phone, emotionally overcome as she spoke to one of our study coordinators. She explained how difficult her life had become, how she dreaded going to work and was terrified about further cognitive deterioration. By the end of the trial, she hoped she would finally see a light at the end of a very dark tunnel. For thirty minutes a day, five days a week for a month, Ayumi navigated her video character along a maze-like river, collecting targets and avoiding obstacles, all with the seriousness of a runner training for a marathon. She was determined to give her brain the opportunity to recover. As time passed, she noticed that her reading material seemed a little less dense and that she was able to recall information, names, and words without too much trouble. It was exciting for her to realize that her brain was evolving, and to see the gradual return of abilities that she thought she had lost forever. "It's like I have my old brain back," she said. "For the first time since I contracted Covid, I feel hopeful."

While our research into EndeavorRx's effectiveness in treating Covid-induced cognitive impairment is still ongoing, some trial participants, like Ayumi, are experiencing positive results. In some cases, physicians have begun to prescribe it for "off label" use to treat cognitive deficits in long Covid and I believe it is worth exploring this possibility. More details can be found at endeavorrx.com.

As of this writing, there are ten registered clinical trials available that focus on cognitive rehabilitation in Covid survivors with cognitive impairment, and a few of them, including the CONTACT Trial, involve neuroplasticity-based restorative training. They can be found at clinicaltrials.gov, a searchable database of privately and publicly funded clinical trials being conducted around the world that is supported by the National Institutes of Health. Such trials often recruit patients locally, although some recruit more widely, even nationally. If you find a trial that might work for you based on eligibility criteria, you can reach out to a study coordinator or perhaps a principal investigator through the provided contact information. It is always a good idea to speak with your doctor or healthcare professional, too.

Brain Training

Of course, clinical trials, while an option for some, are not possible or practical for everyone. There are, however, a variety of other ways that you can access treatments that have the potential to restore and strengthen cognitive function. Some of these involve commercially available brain-training programs, of which perhaps the best known and certainly one of the forerunners is BrainHQ (brainhq.com). Designed by a team of neuroscientists, with eminent neuroscientist and co-inventor of the cochlear implant, Dr. Mike Merzenich, at the helm, BrainHQ offers a suite of individualized brain-training exercises that can be accessed by subscription (there is a limited free option) and played on a computer, tablet, or phone.[11] There are twenty-nine exercises available that work on different areas—including attention, processing speed, memory, and people skills—and an algorithm personalizes the experience, providing structure and order and suggesting which games to play. The software tracks individual progress.

Other similar brain-training options include Peak, Elevate, Lumosity, Happy Neuron, Braingle, Psychology Compass, and Forest. Some commercially available brain-training programs offer coaches, for a fee, to motivate patients and remind them to stay on task.

People around the world have been training their brains long before the emergence of computer programs, and scientific research strongly supports the benefits of activities that keep the brain active. Some options that you may find beneficial include:

- Sudoku
- Scrabble
- Crossword puzzles
- Playing cards
- Learning a foreign language
- Taking up a musical instrument
- Engaging in a new hobby

Activities that involve social engagement can be especially helpful so it can be a good idea to combine brain training with a friend or family member, when possible. It should be noted that not all activities are equally beneficial, and to obtain optimal benefit, activities must involve at least a modest degree of challenge—if they don't stretch you and move you out of your comfort zone, at least a little, you may need to consider trying more difficult options. Improvement is more likely when training is carried out on a regular basis. Some of my patients have set themselves strict schedules that incorporate thirty minutes a day of brain games or word puzzles and, over time, have shown considerable improvement in their cognitive function. Others have a brain workout buddy or someone who holds them accountable to do their daily training.

WHEN MENTAL HEALTH IMPACTS COGNITIVE FUNCTIONING

Over the past couple of years, I've seen cognitive rehabilitation therapy— both compensatory and restorative—bring real change into the daily lives of my patients struggling with long Covid. Sometimes, though, cognitive difficulties are caused not by cognitive deficits but by mental health conditions, and rehabilitation professionals are usually on the lookout for the presence of depression and/or anxiety, which can interfere with cognitive functioning. Time after time, we find that the single greatest barrier to improved cognition is untreated psychological concerns, and that once these issues are identified and effectively addressed, problems with attention, memory, and processing speed often improve. Sometimes, a rehabilitation professional's greatest contribution to their patient's well-being is helping them find the mental health treatment they need.

This was the case with Madison, a Covid survivor with whom I've often consulted. A student at a local university, she struggled to get back on track after coming down with Covid and, by the time I saw her, she was having great difficulty focusing, was rarely attending classes, and was failing the ones that she did manage to get to. She was referred to a speech and language pathologist due to concerns about potential cognitive impairment and was taught a variety of skills that helped with time management and dividing complex tasks into manageable parts. But the thoughtful clinician's most enduring contribution was realizing that Madison had severe depression, new to her after Covid, and assisted her in finding a mental health practitioner. As Madison experienced a remission of her mood-related issues, her cognitive challenges began to improve.

Madison's story is a reminder of the potential limitations of cognitive rehabilitation when other factors are in play, the importance of viewing people through a variety of lenses as opposed to just one, and the value of going to a specialist for help with cognitive impairment as there are treatments available, even if they may be different than initially imagined.

THE IMPORTANCE OF PURSUING TREATMENT

For many years, I've conducted disability examinations at the local VA hospital and during that time I've met countless men and women who have made an indelible impact on me. Often, they served bravely in Iraq or Afghanistan, sometimes across multiple tours, and survived blasts from IED explosions that didn't kill them but contributed to mild traumatic brain injuries that changed the trajectories of their lives. Their cognitive deficits are similar to those I see in my long Covid patients and, in so many cases, treatments were available that could heal and transform but my patients were embarrassed to pursue them, believed they didn't deserve them, or thought they wouldn't work or that their problems would quickly resolve on their own. Sadly, without treatment, over the years, their cognitive deficits led to difficulties holding down jobs, financial struggles, substance use disorders, failed marriages, anger management problems, and alienated children. It didn't have to be that way.

This does not have to be, should not be, *must not be your story.* Cognitive impairment, whether acquired due to a bomb blast or long Covid, is largely treatable. While it may seem as if the path toward recovery is complex, as it can take a referral from a primary care doctor to a neuropsychologist or neurologist and then a referral to an SLP or occupational therapist before rehabilitation can begin, it is worth pursuing. Many people (including doctors) are still unaware that treatment is available for illness-induced cognitive impairment so you may have to be very clear in your goals, specific in mentioning Goal Management Training as an example of a complementary cognitive rehabilitation therapy, or brain training in reference to neuroplasticity-based therapy, and persistent in getting a referral or two if one is not forthcoming. In addition, be sure to track your symptoms of cognitive impairment and the way they affect and impede your daily functioning—referring back to Chapter 2 may be helpful here—and share them with your doctor. The more detail you can provide about what is happening to you and what you need, the easier it will be for a health professional to help you.

The ultimate goal of cognitive rehabilitation is not to increase the number of words you can remember or reduce the speed it takes to connect the dots on a processing-speed test but, rather, to improve functioning in your daily life and get you back on track, whether at work, school, the grocery store, home, or while engaging in hobbies. Research will no doubt clarify questions regarding the impact of rehabilitation on cognitive impairment in those with long Covid but right now a majority of the patients we refer for treatment report experiencing benefits. Whether difficulties first emerged at the beginning of the pandemic or within the past few months, cognitive improvement is possible and attainable. I hope this can be your story, too.

CHAPTER 4

WHEN SADNESS AND STRESS WON'T GO AWAY: Mental Health Challenges in Long Haulers

The beach had always been her happy place, Clara told me, as we sat in my office. She was a relatively new patient and I listened as she described a recent visit to the ocean when her thoughts had turned darker than usual. As the sun disappeared, she had sat in her folding chair, surrounded only by stars and the gentle sounds of lapping waves, and gazed out at the vast expanse of water, wondering what it would be like to swim toward the horizon until she slipped beneath the surface and drowned. It seemed to her a peaceful, even poetic, way to go, to be free of the soul-crushing sadness she had known since losing several jobs, her cognitive ability, and much of her vitality after contracting Covid. "I just feel so low," she said. "All the time."

Clara was caught in the snare of depression, weighted down by a heavy sadness that even robbed her of the desire to break free. Like Clara, many Covid survivors struggle with mental health conditions such as anxiety, depression, PTSD, obsessive-compulsive disorder, and substance use disorders that impact their lives on a daily basis. For some, these may be new, brought on by Covid-19, while for others the virus may have exacerbated preexisting conditions. The reasons for this are not yet clear but one possible biological cause could be dysfunction of the central nervous system, which can contribute to cognitive and psychiatric difficulties. Many Covid survivors who spent time in an ICU develop mental health conditions, such as anxiety and PTSD, brought on by their harrowing hospital experience. In addition, some post-Covid mental health conditions in long haulers can be attributed to lost jobs, financial insecurity, loss of identity, family disruption, traumatic experiences, or the many sudden changes brought on by life with a chronic illness. In far too many cases, people with long Covid are not receiving help because their mental health needs go unrecognized and, more often than not, untreated. In this chapter, I explore various conditions and describe how they might manifest in someone's day-to-day life, helping patients and families look for clues and red flags that could indicate the need for an evaluation, and offer guidance on how to move forward.

Whenever I mention—whether to new acquaintances at a wedding or fellow travelers at the airport—that I'm a psychologist who studies and tends to people with long Covid, I'm often inundated with stories of mental health struggles. I always feel humbled when people share with such raw honesty, and I'm struck each time by the numbers of people navigating mental health conditions after Covid and aware that in my clinic I'm probably witnessing the proverbial tip of the iceberg.

According to both anecdotal and scientific data, the iceberg itself is enormous. To date, more than 22,000 scientific papers have been published on mental health and Covid, capturing, to some degree, the extent of the problem. In likely the largest study to date, a retrospective review published in *Lancet Psychiatry* in 2021 analyzed the medical records of 236,000 patients from the United States who had contracted Covid and found that 33 percent of them had a neuropsychiatric diagnosis six months after their initial infection (46 percent if they had been admitted to an ICU).[1] In another investigation of more than 3,900 individuals evaluating the presence of mental health disorders in long haulers, the most common condition was depression, with 52 percent of Covid survivors meeting criteria for major depressive disorder an average of four months after contracting the virus.[2] People with more-severe initial infections as well as those who were older versus younger were more likely to be depressed.

PTSD also occurs in long haulers at extremely high rates. One 2021 study done in Italy, comprising 381 patients admitted to the hospital with Covid-19, documented that 30.2 percent of patients surviving Covid still had this condition at least four months later.[3] This is a very high percentage—about four times higher than that observed in the general population and slightly higher than is typically reported in combat veterans.

Anxiety affects approximately 22 percent of individuals up to one year after developing Covid-19, according to a large analysis that evaluated results from twenty-seven international studies of more than nine thousand Covid survivors,[4] and while OCD has been studied less extensively than anxiety, depression, and PTSD, one Indian study reported that more than 80 percent of Covid survivors had "new onset" OCD symptoms and reported contamination fears.[5] A study of more than 150,000 patients in the Department of Veterans Affairs healthcare system demonstrated that, when compared to those who had not had Covid-19, individuals testing positive for the virus were 20 percent more likely to develop alcohol-related disorders, and 46 percent more likely to experience suicidal ideation. These kinds of figures are seen across multiple studies.

While risk factors for developing mental health conditions after a Covid infection vary widely, as does severity of illness, several reliable insights have emerged: people with prior mental health histories are especially vulnerable to developing psychiatric problems (including both a recurrence—or exacerbation—of old ones and clinically distinct new ones), people with more-severe acute Covid symptoms generally have more-severe mental health symptoms over time, women seem to be at higher risk for poor mental health outcomes, and symptoms do usually improve. There is no doubt that a wide range of mental health conditions has emerged in epidemic numbers in Covid survivors, and the focus now needs to be on helping people living with long Covid get treatment that can make a huge difference in their quality of life.

AMEERA'S STORY

Fifty-five-year-old Ameera was wracked with feelings of shame, believing she was to blame for contracting Covid during the early days of the pandemic and for the far-reaching problems that had ensued. An extended stay in an intensive care unit with more than a hundred days on extracorporeal membrane oxygenation, an advanced form of life support, had left the family reeling financially, and Ameera, traumatized by her hospital experience, and not feeling well enough to return to her job as a floral designer, now struggled to find a sense of purpose in her life. Her coping mechanisms brought moments of relief but had caused her to gain fifty pounds in six months, rendering her almost unrecognizable. As potato chip bags and ice cream containers littered her kitchen and filled the nook between her couch and chair, she slipped ever deeper into a cycle of shame, hoping, as she dozed off, that tomorrow would be a better day.

Her usually supportive family didn't know what to do, and while their collective hearts were in the right place, they wavered between coaxing, badgering, bullying, and taunting to get Ameera off the couch and moving again. Fueled by well-meaning ignorance, they thought her difficulties were failures of effort and perhaps even character on her part. If she just tried a little harder, they said, with varying degrees of patience, she would soon snap out of the cycle she found herself in. Her sister pointed out how much time had passed since Ameera's hospital discharge and suggested that she should now be hunting for a job she could do from home instead of lounging around eating ice cream.

Ameera's husband was convinced that she would be her old self again once she started working and hovered over her while she applied online to jobs that he suggested. "You'll see!" he said. "You'll thank me later."

Many people simply don't know what symptoms of mental illness are and how they may manifest in someone's life. Unless they have had previous experience with mental health conditions, they may rely on knowledge—often inaccurate—gleaned from television, movies, or social media. This can have most unhelpful consequences. Not long ago, I saw a patient who had one of the more severe cases of PTSD that I had seen in recent years. He was a thoughtful and insightful person, and I was a little puzzled that he hadn't previously sought treatment to deal with the effects of his trauma. His answer? He hadn't experienced the flashbacks that are such a common feature of popular PTSD portrayals, and so had assumed that he didn't suffer from the syndrome. In reality, flashbacks are a relatively uncommon symptom of PTSD.

MENTAL HEALTH CHALLENGES IN DAILY LIFE

Just as cognitive difficulties due to long Covid can make it challenging to get through a typical day, so, too, can mental health struggles, as they often impact multiple aspects of a person's life. My aim here is to identify indicators of mental health conditions in real-life situations so that you can consider whether you—or a loved one—might need to seek treatment. You may recognize yourself, or family members, in the descriptions that follow and may want to self-diagnose. At that point, as I outline in the chapter, I recommend that you seek help from a healthcare professional to determine if you could benefit from treatment.

Anxiety

Anxiety impacts people in all kinds of situations, especially during a pandemic, but it moves from being a nuisance ("I'm so stressed because my car won't start, and I'll be late!") to a clinical concern when it becomes overwhelming, long lasting, and hard to manage. Among the various manifestations of anxiety, the most common is Generalized Anxiety Disorder (GAD), which is diagnosed when someone experiences at least six months of excessive, disproportionate worry about everyday issues. While you might consider it reasonable for someone with long Covid to be worried about their life, health, and future, it is important to be aware of when anxiety is interfering with, and limiting, life. Common manifestations of GAD in long haulers include:

- Having problems coping with uncertainty and worrying about potential negative outcomes that are unknown and can't be controlled—to the extent that it can be very hard to enjoy anything. Whenever Adam, one of my patients, thinks about making plans for his future, he focuses on scenarios of failure (*I might not pass the exam so what's the point in taking it? Maybe everyone on that dating app will reject me*), so he stays home, safe from adverse interactions with the world, but not really able to do much at all.

- Fixating on worst-case scenarios, often known as catastrophizing. This can be especially common in people living with long Covid who may feel that they will never get better or return to any semblance of their life prior to Covid.

- Creating "what ifs" that may never happen such as, *What if I catch Covid again and am unable to work? What if the economy crashes and my 401(k) is wiped out? What if, having survived Covid, I die of cancer? What if my dog's collar breaks and she runs onto the highway?*

- One worry leads to many worries. I find that many of my patients have what might be thought of as "sessions" of anxiety that stem from one thought, say, feeling stress about an upcoming medical appointment, which then expands to concern about insurance reimbursements, about financial instability, paying for college, their kids' grades, not being a good enough parent, until they are overwhelmed by an onslaught of global anxiety.

- Avoiding activities, responsibilities, or people. This may begin on a small scale such as one missed class (*I don't want to be called on as I didn't do the reading*) and then escalate, each new avoidance building on the last (*The professor will be mad because I missed the last two classes so I can't go today*) until the missed classes turn into a dropped course, which comes with additional anxiety. This anxiety may generalize into avoiding all emails or phone calls in case they contain stressful information, which can lead to bigger problems down the road.

- Suffering physical symptoms such as sweating, upset stomach, breathlessness, and headaches. Be aware if instances of feeling off or not quite well occur frequently, especially before activities, events, or responsibilities. While the symptoms are completely real and should not be dismissed, they may be rooted in anxiety.

Another anxiety disorder affecting long haulers is panic disorder, in which people experience panic attacks — extremely frightening episodes that develop rapidly. During a panic attack, which typically reaches a peak over several minutes, people experience intense physical and psychological symptoms that can include sweating, shortness of breath, chest pain, a sense of "unreality" or being detached, heart racing, a sense of impending doom, and fear of losing control. Panic attacks, which often develop with no warning, are experienced by Covid survivors in a variety of situations, such as:

- After learning they or their family members have been exposed to Covid.
- On finding out that their PCP no longer sees patients using telehealth and realizing that they will have to meet in person.
- When experiencing physical sensations like shortness of breath, which may stimulate anxious thoughts about symptoms worsening.
- After watching the news or going online and hearing about upsetting events.

Depression

A common condition in survivors of Covid, depression can take various forms, with the most prevalent type known as major depressive disorder. It is diagnosed when key symptoms, such as a depressed mood and a loss of interest in activities, are present every day for at least two weeks. Be aware of the following symptoms and behaviors, which are often seen in long haulers and may indicate the presence of depression:

- Anhedonia, a technical term that refers to the inability or reduced ability to feel pleasure, can show up as a lack of interest in activities that used to be a source of enjoyment. One of my patients is an avid golfer and usually looks forward to watching the Masters Tournament with as much excitement as I anticipate the Super Bowl. Every year, he eagerly awaits the event, even taking vacation days so he can view it live in his man cave. But not this year. When the tournament took place in April, he didn't even turn on his television—a sign that suggested to his wife and family that the low mood he had experienced since recovering from Covid was perhaps more significant than they'd thought and that led him to seek mental health treatment.

- Intense feelings of worthlessness or guilt, often accompanied by self-blame. For many long haulers, these emotions can be heightened by being out of work, or unable to participate in family events or engage in activities that were once a source of satisfaction. Ameera struggled with such feelings, blaming herself for catching Covid and bringing on subsequent difficulties for herself and her family. Often family members can unintentionally exacerbate these feelings.

- Sad, empty, or hopeless feelings that occur during most of every day. These can exacerbate difficulties with self-motivation. Some of my patients report feeling that everything is pointless and so why make the huge effort to do something? In these cases, it may seem as if someone with depression is not trying hard enough, or at all.

- Sleep issues, including insomnia (trouble either falling asleep, staying asleep, or waking up too early and being unable to go back to sleep) and sleeping too much. These can intensify feelings of exhaustion and contribute to a lack of energy, which can, in turn, make it difficult for someone to handle commitments—or daily life.

- Problems with concentration and decision-making. These fairly common symptoms are often overlooked or dismissed but they can undermine a person's ability to function in many areas. Often, they can be challenging to diagnose because although they may reflect depression, they could be symptoms of cognitive dysfunction, so prevalent in those with long Covid. One of my patients found it almost impossible to focus on his sales job after contracting Covid but when he was treated for other symptoms of depression his capacity to concentrate returned.

- Recurring thoughts of death or suicide, which may, in more worrisome cases, involve an active desire to end one's life. In other instances, these may involve vague thoughts that *family and friends would be better off without me* or, perhaps, that it might be desirable to fall asleep at night and never wake up. Signs of suicidal ideation include talking about wanting to die or to not be alive, making comments such as, "Well, that won't matter because I won't be around for it," researching suicide methods, talking about being a burden on others, withdrawing from social connections, giving away possessions, making a will. I provide more details later in the chapter on how to respond.

Post-Traumatic Stress Disorder (PTSD)

PTSD is a relatively new name for a disorder with a long history. Prviously known as soldier's heart, battle fatigue, or shell shock—reflecting an early belief that it developed exclusively in response to combat—we now know that it occurs as a reaction to a traumatic event (or ongoing events and experiences) that causes someone's whole system to feel threatened. Our body's automatic survival mechanisms spring into action, which can be useful in the moment but less so when an intense, frequent, or prolonged reaction lingers in the body and resurfaces later. Defined by the DSM-5 as "having direct or indirect exposure to a traumatic event, followed by symptoms in four categories: intrusion, avoidance, negative changes in thoughts and mood, and changes in arousal and reactivity," PTSD can unfold in the lives of survivors of Covid-19 in various ways. Symptoms and behaviors, which can overlap with symptoms of anxiety and depression, include:

- Intrusive and persistent memories of being acutely ill with Covid-19, which can lead someone to reexperience their illness and the accompanying emotions (fear, sadness, loneliness, etc.). Memories may appear to arise out of nowhere or can be activated by sights, sounds, or smells. One of my patients described feeling unpleasant emotions every time he thought about his ICU diary, a handwritten booklet created for him by a nurse that chronicled the details of his hospital stay, many of which he didn't remember because he had been sedated. These helpful diaries are increasingly employed in the care of critically ill patients to provide a factual narrative of their hospital stay, which can then replace the sometimes terrifying, often delirium-induced, thoughts and memories of the ICU that can torment them for months, or years, afterward. The diaries, usually read with patients on or after discharge, have been shown to be effective in reducing the risk of depression and anxiety and improving quality of life, but my patient was reluctant to engage. Even the thought of reading about his critical illness brought back uncomfortable emotions and memories.
- Avoidance of medical clinics, hospitals, and medical procedures, even important ones. Patients, especially those who were

hospitalized or in the ICU due to Covid, are often reluctant to return to places they associate — either directly or indirectly — with physically and emotionally painful aspects of their illness. I've had patients request telehealth visits as they believe that returning to the hospital where they were treated will provoke intense feelings of distress. Recently, a patient, who spent more than two months in an ICU after contracting Covid and now has severe PTSD, shared a story with me. One of his friends was recovering in a local hospital after a bad car accident, and my patient wanted to visit — but the thought of going back to a hospital was terrifying. It took him several days to ready himself to see his friend in the critical care unit and, though he was proud he was able to do this, his voice shook as he recounted the significant anguish he had felt. Avoidance, like most symptoms, exists on a spectrum; some individuals are better able to push back against their fears, while others orient their lives around finding ways to evade unpleasant reminders. Be aware that any degree of avoidance could be a sign that something is awry.

- Intense, future-oriented concerns about the possibility of contracting Covid-19 again that go beyond "normal" worry. Many Covid survivors experience intense panic if they learn that a family member has tested positive, that a new variant has been found, or that local Covid prevalence rates are on the rise.

- A phobic-like focus on germs, hygiene, or cleanliness that leads to isolation, far beyond what is typical, even during a pandemic. Some of my patients have hunkered down in their homes, living hermit-like lives, and while such an approach may decrease the likelihood of contracting Covid-19 again, intense isolation can lead to the development of other problems, such as depression.

- Negative changes in thoughts and mood, often reflected in fiercely critical patterns of self-blame. I've had numerous patients upbraid themselves for catching Covid, harshly lashing out and calling themselves names, speaking in ways they would never speak to others, using words and phrases laced with negativity.

- Hypervigilance, expressed through intense preoccupation with and constant monitoring of one's health. This might include frequent checks of temperature, oxygen levels, and heart rate. There could also be a need to test regularly for Covid, even when symptoms are not present and recent exposure is unlikely.

- Sleep difficulties can occur, especially if intrusive memories have appeared in dreams or nightmares, as there may be a reluctance to open oneself up to the possibility of reoccurrence by falling asleep. Many of my patients report extremely vivid dreams of their experiences of being acutely ill with Covid and, in some cases, in the minutes and hours after waking up, they struggle to separate these dreams from reality.

- Intense guilt over the possibility that one might have spread Covid-19 and brought on the illness or even the death of others.

Obsessive-Compulsive Disorder (OCD)

People with obsessive-compulsive disorder have recurring obsessions (unwanted, intrusive, and often upsetting thoughts, images, or urges) that usually lead them to engage in compulsions (repetitive behaviors, rituals, or thoughts intended to decrease obsessions and the distress they cause). Be on the lookout for the following symptoms of OCD in people with long Covid:

Obsessions

- Unwanted thoughts of harming oneself or others, often unintentionally. These could include repetitive thoughts that you fatally infected someone with Covid-19 or that you might accidentally run someone over with your car.

- Doubts that you've been vaccinated for Covid (even though you were) or fears that you have Covid, even though multiple test

results show you are negative. As a reminder, doubt is a core feature of OCD and is expressed through countless examples,
Covid-related or not—e.g., someone cooks eggs for breakfast
before leaving for work, then worries all day that they may not
have turned off the stove.

- Thoughts about acting inappropriately in public—e.g., cough-
ing on someone or yelling "I have Covid" in a crowd. Acting in
inappropriate ways in public is a frequent fear of mine, and in
recent months I've developed a particular worry about saying the
word *bomb* while in an airport. Such fears, which people worry
they will act on, are an often-terrifying feature of OCD and,
unfortunately, they can lead to isolation and avoidance of social
situations.

- Fears that feel like urges to say something sexually provocative,
perhaps to a colleague on a Zoom call, or relentless anxieties that
you may have done so, which may lead you to check with another
colleague or, if you have a recording, rewatching it multiple
times to convince yourself that you didn't say or do anything
inappropriate.

- Worries that your neighbor with Covid-19 won't recover unless
you pray the same prayer at the same time every night or carry
out a similar ritual.

It can be hard for others to recognize obsessions in someone else. However, if someone has OCD you might notice that they repeatedly ask
you for reassurance that they haven't harmed you or wronged you in
any way. This could include reassurance that is impossible to give, such
as that everything is going to be fine or that you will remain healthy.
They may tell you that they have unwanted thoughts racing through
their mind or ask you to sit with them as they don't want to be alone
with their ruminations. You may observe that they are constantly on
their phone, scrolling, texting, watching videos, or playing games,

which could be an attempt to distract themselves from a stressful internal monologue. Growing dependency on substances such as alcohol or drugs can be a sign of an attempt at self-medication.

Compulsions

- Developing a new preoccupation with personal cleanliness, for instance, beginning to take frequent daily baths and multiple long showers. Fear of contamination appears to be the most common OCD symptom since the beginning of the pandemic.[6] I've had patients engage in compulsive handwashing. Often, after washing their hands a dozen or more times, they bump their hand on something while leaving the kitchen or bathroom and have to begin the entire process again.
- Cleanliness in the environment. This includes wiping down groceries and mail, sanitizing countertops, door handles, and remote controls.
- Repeating the same phrase or sentence in your mind or the same behavior—e.g., taking rapid Covid tests repeatedly just to make sure you are Covid negative, or fixating on words with five letters and saying them over and over.
- Staying home as a way of making sure that you do not do or say the wrong thing in public.
- Hoarding, including items such as cleaning products and supplies, and masks for fear of running out. Keeping greetings cards and gifts out of worry that, if you don't, something bad might happen to the person who sent or gave them.

When I developed OCD in 2018, there were relatively few overt signs, partly because I struggle with "Pure O"—which involves few obvious compulsions—but I knew immediately that something was wrong. In the early days of my illness, I noticed new thoughts that were strange, unfamiliar, and disturbing. Two examples stand out: the fear that I might pull a fire alarm every time I saw one; and the worry that I might deliberately scrape someone's car with my key whenever I walked through the parking lot at work. As I reflect on this season, I remember hurrying past the red alarms, my hands stuffed deep in pockets, and I recall the jagged feel of my car keys as I held them tight inside my fist as I navigated through the parking lot. Soon, these weird but innocuous thoughts gave way to far more disturbing urges, which ultimately led me to discuss my concerns with a psychologist.

Sometimes, behaviors related to OCD may not be obvious to others, especially when they occur deep inside someone's mind, and if you are experiencing unwanted and persistent thoughts and engaging in compulsive behaviors, you don't need confirmation from a family member or friend that something is amiss. It is time to get help.

Psychosis

Psychosis refers to a condition that causes someone to have disordered thoughts and perceptions that lack a basis in reality, making it difficult for them to determine what is real and what is not. Of the syndromes described in this chapter, it is clearly the rarest, and though emerging literature suggests that it is more common in Covid survivors than in the general US population, limited data about its prevalence exists. In my first twenty-seven years of practice as a therapist, I encountered only one patient who had developed psychosis, an engineer in New York City who had reached out to me for guidance, while in the last year I have treated or consulted with five. My observations are supported by recent literature, largely in the form of individual case studies, suggesting that "Covid-19 psychosis," as some propose it should be called, is indeed a phenomenon, although a relatively rare one and with more questions than answers. Studies to date paint a picture of a condition that predominantly affects middle-aged men, most with no psychiatric history whatsoever. Its symptoms, which wax and wane and usually resolve eventually, result in diagnoses such as Acute Psychotic Disorder or Psychotic Disorder Not Otherwise Specified.

Be aware of the following symptoms:

- Hallucinations involving feeling, hearing, or, most commonly, seeing things that are not there. In my clinical experience, these are among the most typical features of Covid-19 psychosis. One of my patients, with no prior history of psychosis, came to see me when he started experiencing hallucinations on at least a weekly basis, usually visual and involving fleeting images of a woman dressed in old-fashioned attire, though auditory on occasion.
- Delusions, often of a paranoid or persecutory nature. These are deeply held beliefs despite evidence to the contrary and may include the bizarre (your dog is secretly the King of Spain) or the non-bizarre (your neighbors have set up video cameras and are spying on you for the government).
- Disorganized speech, including speaking incoherently, changing topics rapidly and in an illogical way, and giving answers that don't correspond to the questions being asked.
- Apathy and listlessness. Psychosis causes significant changes in behavior and often manifests as apathy in people who are usually responsible, motivated, and energetic. I recently consulted with a patient who ran a successful lawn-mowing business and was well known in his small town for his dynamism and work ethic. When he suddenly became unconcerned about maintaining his fleet of lawn mowers, responding to the many messages his customers left, or balancing his books, it was clear that something was going on.
- Catatonic behavior, often marked by signs of stupor, in which patients cannot speak, move, or respond and often appear rigid. These symptoms, while common in people with psychotic disorders, seem to be rarely reported in Covid survivors with psychosis.

Substance Use Disorders (SUDs)

Substance use disorders are mental health disorders that impact wide-ranging areas of functioning and involve a person's inability to control their use of substances, whatever they might be (alcohol, drugs, prescription and non-prescription medication). They can range from mild to severe and often occur along with other mental health conditions, including anxiety, depression, PTSD, and OCD. According to the *DSM-5*, an SUD diagnosis needs eleven different symptoms to be present, and although a full description of these is beyond the scope of this chapter, be aware of these key symptoms:

- Using a substance to handle anxiety or to destress.
- Using more of a substance or taking a substance for a longer period of time than you're meant to.
- Using a substance to try to change a mood or sustain a mood, perhaps drinking to keep on feeling happy or to numb one's pain.
- Desiring to stop or reduce the use of a substance but finding that you're unable to.
- Reducing or ceasing your involvement in important roles or activities and functioning less effectively because of substance use.
- Continuing to use substances, even when it is harmful or puts you in danger.
- Experiencing withdrawal symptoms that can be temporarily alleviated by using more substances.
- Being willing to compromise relationships through lying, stealing, etc., in pursuit of the next drink or the next high.

Substance use disorders have increased significantly since the start of the pandemic, both among people with long Covid, and in society more generally, with one study reporting that 31 percent of people have increased their alcohol consumption and 29 percent have increased their drug use.

Such increases are likely fueled by mental health concerns (e.g., people feel anxiety and drink to try to relieve it), financial stress, and other pressures but may be made worse by current work-from-home situations where individuals lack the accountability they previously had when they had to report to an office. As one pundit said, "You can't smell alcohol on someone's breath on a Zoom call." People frequently feel unsafe or ashamed talking about their substance use, whether alcohol or, even more so, drugs.

HOW TO SUPPORT SOMEONE WITH SYMPTOMS OF MENTAL ILLNESS

Mental health conditions can present in confusing and complex ways for both the person experiencing the illness and their family and friends. It can be difficult to understand why someone may be behaving in a certain way or even to accept that their symptoms constitute an illness. Ameera's family loved her greatly and yet their responses to her new behaviors—lying on the couch and eating comfort foods—were neither kind nor helpful. Instead, they added to her feelings of shame and hopelessness.

When someone exhibits signs of mental illness, it is important to show compassion while encouraging them to get treatment. In my experience, nagging people with mental illness to change their behavior results in worse outcomes when compared to offering positive support, so be aware of the way you are interacting. Try to avoid the following:

- *Minimizing*—e.g., "I know you're worried about things but trust me, I don't think it's that big of a deal. Everything will be just fine."
- *Moralizing*—e.g., "Ameera, if you'd just stop eating all that junk food, you'd feel a lot better. No wonder you want to lie around all day. Let's get you eating salads and sleeping at the proper time."
- *Spiritualizing*—e.g., "Honey, if you start living for God, I think He'll take the desire for alcohol away—you just have to surrender."

- *Blaming*—e.g., "If you had just talked to your doctor about this a few months ago like I suggested, I don't think you would be in this situation now."
- *Shaming*—e.g., "What are my mom and dad, let alone my partners at work and the neighbors, going to say if we have to admit you to the psych ward? That's the last place you need to go, Sharon—that would be a major embarrassment."

My long Covid patients often tell me of the destructive words their family members or friends have said while trying to be helpful. They contrast starkly with the responses that are needed. Let's explore more effective ways of relating:

- *Listen carefully/nonjudgmentally.* Don't be quick to interject your opinions or to frame things as "good" or "bad." Repeat back the things you think you've heard, to communicate that you understand. "What I'm hearing you say is that you're sure your boss is about to fire you."
- *Empathize.* Even if you've never experienced similar symptoms, you can likely identify with what it's like to feel sad, or down, or out of control. Relate from an empathic place of understanding. "That's sounds really difficult. I'm sorry you're going through this."
- *Offer honest feedback if given the chance.* Frequently, family members or friends are asked by patients if they have noticed any changes in their personalities or behaviors and if they have any concerns. If you've been asked this question, think of it as a privilege. Step up and share kindly and honestly. If you've observed issues of concern, highlight how they have impacted you. Often, these sincere accounts help people understand the reality of their problems and result in people seeking help.
- *Don't overreact.* It often takes an act of great courage for someone to be vulnerable about their mental health concerns, and

meeting such disclosures with bewilderment, disbelief, or fear can cause people to retreat and shut down a potential conversation. Recently, I was having lunch with a new friend at a popular restaurant near the medical center and, in the middle of an honest conversation, I decided to share that I had OCD. She listened, nodded her head, thanked me for sharing, and kept on eating, gently normalizing this and showing me that it wasn't too big an admission for her to handle. May we all relate with such grace.

- *Decrease stigma by sharing your own stories.* Not long ago, I met with a patient who clearly suffered from depression. He was in counseling but had made little headway and his therapist had suggested that he consider taking an antidepressant. He explained that he was resistant to do this. I offered my own story, that I, too, had been on the fence about psychiatric medication but had reluctantly agreed to take Prozac and found it very helpful. This simple truth—that other people relied on medication as part of their mental health toolkit—gave him an extra piece of information to consider. Later, he told me he'd decided to give medication a try.

- *Offer help in finding support rather than try to diagnose.* You're likely not a mental health specialist, and acting as if you are will usually engender defensiveness. Displaying a willingness to provide support, however, is helpful. Support could mean being available to join a doctor's visit or researching different therapists.

GETTING TREATMENT

You should now be better able to understand if you or a family member may be struggling with mental illness that would benefit from treatment. What should you do? Can certain signs be ignored? When should they be taken seriously? And what are the red flags that should result in immediate treatment?

Urgent: Immediate Action Required

A key insight is that all mental health symptoms are *not* created equal. Some bring minimal disruption to a person's life while others are urgent concerns. Of these, the most important are symptoms that impact personal safety (such as suicidal ideation), those that impair a patient's reality testing (the ability to know what is real), and those that, if untreated, would likely lead to significant health, financial, and/or legal concerns (such as substance use).

Suicidal Ideation

While many people have contemplated suicide at one point or another in their lives, or thought that they no longer wished to be alive, it is concerning if you or someone you know has persistent thoughts of wanting to die. It is especially vital that you seek support when two components are combined: 1) a desire ("I would like to end my life") and 2) a specific plan ("I'm going to jump off the Mackinaw Bridge on Monday night"). When suicidal thoughts are enduring, worsening, or involve the development of a specific plan, it is time to get immediate help from a professional by calling a local or national suicide hotline (call or text 988), going to the emergency room, or calling 911 and stating it is a psychiatric emergency.

Active Psychosis

When medical professionals think of the entire range of possible psychiatric symptoms, signs of psychosis, especially if they develop suddenly in people without a prior history, represent the severe end of the spectrum. Rapidly emerging symptoms—including hallucinations or strikingly paranoid or delusional thinking—can impair a person's ability to function and leave them vulnerable to harm. They may also reflect underlying processes in the brain, such as encephalitis. Either way, signs of psychosis always require urgent medical attention that may include a visit to an emergency room or an urgent care.

Substance Use

Substance use can take many forms, including alcohol, marijuana, prescription medicines, methamphetamine, cocaine, and opiates, sometimes used separately and sometimes together. While treatment of substance use is always important, it becomes urgent in these situations:

- In the case of alcohol, when drinking moves from being infrequent and under control to being frequent and out of control (e.g., bingeing, resulting in blackouts).
- With drug use, when occasional experimentation becomes regular use.
- When substance use becomes a way to cope with difficult emotions and feelings.
- When an attempt has been made to stop using substances but has failed.
- When substance use gets in the way of daily functioning.
- When physical or psychological cravings are present.
- When personality changes are apparent.

As with other conditions, the right place to start is a discussion with your PCP, who can help you find a referral for treatment that may include a 12-step program (Alcoholics Anonymous or something similar), a referral to a mental health professional, or, depending on the severity of symptoms, a rehabilitation facility. If you don't have a primary care provider, you could find a local 12-step meeting or, if you are ill or experiencing withdrawal symptoms, you could go to the ER.

Important: Action Required

Some symptoms may not represent a five-alarm fire and don't call for an immediate trip to the ER, but that doesn't mean they aren't important or don't need to be quickly addressed. Many symptoms require professional attention and should not be overlooked as their presence means they are already impairing someone's quality of life or have the potential to do so. How can you tell when these symptoms should be addressed?

Persistent and Worsening

Mental health symptoms can be evaluated by many criteria but I'm going to introduce two — how long have they persisted, and if they are increasing in frequency or intensity. Have you grappled with feeling sad for a few days or have your feelings lingered for months? Are you having unwanted thoughts about your time in the ICU every two or three days now instead of every two or three weeks? Have the symptoms remained the same, perhaps very mild (you notice intrusive thoughts and then you shake them off), or does it seem like they are getting worse (the intrusive thoughts are constantly present)?

Functionally Disruptive

Sigmund Freud once wrote, "Love and work are the cornerstones of our humanness." Building on this idea, one way to determine if mental health issues need to be addressed is to ask how much they are impacting functioning in these two primary areas — are they affecting your relationships and/or your work (or school or community work, etc.)? Are you often short-tempered and irritable with your spouse or your children or have you disengaged completely from the group text with old high school friends? Are you so preoccupied with the thoughts rumbling in your head that you are increasingly ignoring the people around you? Are you late for meetings? Do you find that you don't care if you do a good job on projects? Are you too anxious to go to class? Have you started to take days off because you can't face your responsibilities? Are you having to push through a hangover from the previous evening of drinking? Is it hard for you to muster the energy to get out of bed in the morning?

A Change in Functioning

A crucial factor in determining whether symptoms need attention is whether they represent a "change" from normal functioning. About fifteen years ago, I saw a combat veteran at a VA clinic. Recently discharged, he was only a few years removed from meritorious service in the Battle of Fallujah, one of the bloodiest battles of Operation Enduring Freedom. I noted that he was alert and on edge, scanning the office and putting his chair in the corner, and assumed that his hypervigilance was a relatively new problem that stemmed from spending most of his deployment in a combat zone. He advised me that these attributes weren't recent arrivals. "I grew up on the South Side of Chicago," he said. "In the Robert Taylor Homes. I learned to watch my back at an early age. If you didn't, you'd get yourself killed. I've always been like this." Some Covid survivors with symptoms of anxiety, depression, and even PTSD have "always been like this,"—that is, their symptoms don't represent a departure from symptoms they've lived with for much of their lives. For such patients, treatment is an individual decision; if they have long-standing symptoms and are functioning well, treatment may not be crucial. However, if symptoms and behaviors represent a change, and are associated with functional difficulties, this is an important red flag suggesting it is time to seek help.

WHEN TO MONITOR SYMPTOMS

In the world of cancer care, an important concept is "watchful waiting," defined by the National Cancer Institute as "closely watching a patient's condition but not giving treatment unless symptoms appear or change."[7] This approach is relevant in the mental health arena as well. Using a watchful-waiting model, patients and their families may notice certain areas of possible concern but decide not to act on these unless things get worse. Consider the following examples:

- Occasional nightmares of traumatic events that happened while in the hospital. They are upsetting but infrequent and they only occur during times of intense stress, typically once every one or two months.
- Feelings of low mood and hopelessness that seem to ebb and flow but don't get in the way of daily living.
- Feelings of mild panic that occur when you compare your pre-Covid activity level to your current level. These symptoms happen infrequently, and you view them as a nuisance as they don't impact your daily life.

If symptoms were to get worse, become more frequent, or interfere with daily functioning, it would be time to consider talking to your PCP.

THERAPY AS A VALUABLE RESOURCE

If you are not struggling with a mental health condition, therapy is not usually necessary. However, if you have the time, energy, and resources, finding a professional you can talk to, who will support and validate your experience, is likely always going to be valuable and something that few long haulers would regret.

When I was in graduate school, participation in psychotherapy was a program requirement; every student had to see an individual psychotherapist once a week for at least one year. I loved it. In my first session, I started talking and the next thing I remember is my psychologist looking at his watch and telling me that he would see me in a week. I talked for the entire session, as I did for many sessions to come. I'm very verbal but I must admit I wasn't aware that I had so much to say and so many complicated emotions to express. We spent long hours processing my feelings of being a failure, my frequent expectations of being abandoned by people in my life, my reluctance to engage in conflict, and my belief that if people placed their faith in me, I'd eventually find a way to let them down.

I came to understand the distortions in my thinking, the relentless ways that I criticized myself, and the complicated dynamics that had shaped me, and that shape all of us. It was helpful and, as my wife will happily attest, even transformative, allowing me to understand my internal processes in new and liberating ways, to live a life of vulnerability and openness, and to make sustained changes that persist to this day. While it was probably not absolutely necessary — meaning that I was functioning at a high enough level without it — it was hugely beneficial in my relationships and my work. Even without a mental health diagnosis, you may find therapy helpful for you, too.

NEXT STEPS: GETTING HELP

Once you have recognized that you or someone you know may have a mental health condition (or perhaps more than one), it is time to begin the process of seeking help. The best place to start is with your primary care physician or, as described in Chapter 1, with a post-Covid clinic. For some people, who may be ambivalent about seeking treatment, this first step may seem easier to take than reaching out to a mental health professional directly. While PCPs are not specialists in mental health care and vary widely in the depth of their knowledge, they are usually open to having conversations with patients about mental health concerns. Often these conversations take place during regular checkups, but patients can — and should, if necessary — schedule appointments solely for the purpose of talking about issues such as anxiety, depression, or any other challenges they are facing. It is helpful to prepare for an appointment (as described in Chapter 1) in order to give the doctor a clear understanding of your symptoms and the way they are affecting your life, and to be able to ask questions you may have.

At the appointment, after listening to your concerns, your doctor may conduct screening tests, roughly analogous to the cognitive screening tests described in Chapter 2—particularly for symptoms of depression and anxiety and substance use.

Common screening tools include:

- Patient Health Questionnaire-9 (PHQ-9), a nine-item form that evaluates the presence of symptoms of depression and their severity.
- Generalized Anxiety Disorder Scale–7 (GAD-7), a seven-item questionnaire that assesses anxiety.
- Hospital Anxiety and Depression Scale (HADS), a fourteen-item tool used to screen for anxiety and depression in inpatient and outpatient medical settings.
- Alcohol Use Disorders Identification Test (AUDIT), a ten-question tool developed by the World Health Organization that evaluates alcohol-related problems.
- Primary Care PTSD Screen (PC-PTSD-5), a five-item screening tool designed for general use. It is less common for PCPs to screen for PTSD (though it is standard practice at Department of Veterans Affairs hospitals and clinics where 9 million veterans receive regular healthcare, including primary care).

These various screening tests are widely known as self-report tools, meaning that they rely on a patient's answers as opposed to the interpretation of clinicians. Frequently, scoring in a particular range on one of these tests—known as a clinical range—will result in a referral.

After evaluating your symptoms, some PCPs may offer to prescribe medication—and oversee symptom management—but this usually only happens in cases where symptoms are very mild or mild—or in cases where the PCP has specialized experience. In most cases, they will refer patients to a mental health professional, usually one of the following:

Clinical Psychologist

Clinical psychologists are licensed mental health professionals who have completed doctoral training (usually a PhD or a PsyD) in clinical psychology and received extensive and highly specialized training in the diagnosis and treatment of a wide range of mental health conditions. They are typically skilled in the assessment of mental illness and provide various kinds of psychotherapy, depending on the needs of their patients. While some are generalists (that is, they treat most conditions), others have specialties, too, and can work with patients with particular needs, e.g., anxiety disorders and chronic health conditions like cancer, spinal cord injuries, HIV-AIDS, trauma, etc. Finding a professional with a specific specialty can be more difficult in rural areas, though telemedicine is proving increasingly helpful.

Clinical Social Worker

Master's-level professionals with expertise in treating a variety of mental health conditions, clinical social workers are often particularly adept at connecting patients to community resources and advocating for crucial support that other mental health providers may overlook, including housing, affordable access to care, legal services, disability, etc.

Employee Assistance Program (EAP)

Many workplaces offer mental health support through an employee assistance program—widely known as an EAP—as a benefit to employees. If you work for a medium- or large-size employer, an EAP of some kind is probably available to you. Mental health providers of various kinds, with diverse levels of experience and wide-ranging types of training, can provide psychological services as part of an EAP program. These confidential services usually comprise a few counseling sessions (three to five) that provide a stopgap while patients find a therapist they can see over a longer period of time.

Mental Health Counselor

Mental health counselors are licensed master's-level professionals who have received training in the treatment of mental health issues. They provide therapy to patients and develop treatment plans, but they may work with less clinically complex patients than psychologists or psychiatrists. While the scope of their clinical practice may be more limited, there are far more mental health counselors than psychologists, and appointments with them can often be made more readily.

Marriage and Family Therapist (MFT)

These master's-level mental health professionals have unique training in family systems therapy, in which individual issues are looked at in the context of couples and families. The effects of long Covid often reverberate from individuals to couples to entire families, and MFTs may be uniquely qualified to help heal relational ruptures that may occur. I discuss long Covid as a family problem in more detail in Chapter 10.

Psychiatrist/Psychiatric Nurse Practitioner

Psychiatrists are medical doctors (MD or DO), and psychiatric nurse practitioners (PNP) are advanced nurses who specialize in the treatment of mental health disorders. They are uniquely qualified to address and understand issues related to the intersection between physical and psychological concerns and help patients determine whether their conditions have a biological basis. While some psychiatrists and PNPs perform psychotherapy, their primary expertise is in the use of medication to manage a full array of psychiatric conditions. Psychiatrists can also prescribe device-based treatments that may be effective when more conventional approaches haven't worked. These include transcranial magnetic stimulation, electroconvulsive therapy, and deep brain stimulation and are discussed more fully in Chapter 5.

In some cases you may be referred to a mental health professional who, after meeting with you, may find it appropriate to refer you to someone else, either instead of them (when more specialized treatment would be useful) or in addition to them (some patients see a psychiatrist, too, when medication is part of a treatment plan).

AMEERA'S STORY

Earlier in this chapter, we left my patient, Ameera, struggling with her mental health, locked in a cycle of shame about having contracted Covid, and trying to manage her sadness and self-loathing by loading up on comfort food, which, inevitably, spiraled her into continuing shame cycles. After several difficult months, Ameera went to her PCP for her annual checkup and, as part of the appointment, mentioned the reason for her weight gain. Her PCP nodded and asked, "Could you tell me more?" Ameera's story flooded out. Covid, the ICU, the terrible months that followed, her family's lack of understanding, the fruitless job search, the lack of meaning in anything anymore. When Ameera stopped talking, the doctor said gently, "I'm sorry you've been feeling that way. I'm glad you're telling me now so that we can get some help for you. I'm wondering if you may have depression. First, let's do a couple of screening tests, and then I'll help you with a referral." Ameera was surprised. "I have an illness that's making me feel like this?" she asked. "I thought I was just tired still. And sad about my life."

"Those things are part of the illness," said the doctor. "But you don't have to keep on feeling this way. There are many treatments available."

Recently Ameera made her way to one of my colleagues and was diagnosed with major depressive disorder. She is currently beginning to make progress through participation in weekly psychotherapy, which is giving her a sense of control over her situation, helping her understand and change the distorted thoughts that contribute to her depression, and fostering in her the belief that she can make changes in her life. One of the most important elements of her treatment has been her understanding and acknowledgment that she is not to blame for the way she feels or for her behavior. From this foundation, she is working on getting better.

Mental health conditions are both common in Covid survivors and frequently under- or untreated. The key to moving forward is to recognize symptoms, to understand how devastating and debilitating an invisible illness can be, and to start the process of treatment. In the next chapter, I'll outline various options for treatment for many different conditions common in long haulers.

THE ONLY WAY AROUND IS THROUGH: Seeking Solutions for Mental Health Issues and Finding the Courage to Pursue Them

Like many other Midwesterners, I grew up fishing. Some of my earliest memories involve sitting on a creekbank, a pole in my hand, and a red-and-white bobber floating on almost stagnant water, waiting for a fish to bite. As I got older, I was excited to move from fishing with worms to using lures, the artificial baits of various kinds that entice elusive fish. I spent countless hours and many of my parents' dollars at our local store, Chopps Bait Shop, just a tiny cottage, really, but filled to the brim with crankbaits, jigs, spoons, and spinners of all kinds, some muted in color and some bright, some big, some small, some designed to float, and others to sink. When I first surveyed the many options available to me, I had no idea where to start. I knew what I wanted to catch, a huge trophy fish, but I was completely unsure of how to go about it, until one day the man behind the counter suggested I try a Rapala, a slender crankbait that moved in the water like an injured minnow. This, he said, was the right bait to catch a lunker, and not long after, I was hoisting my first largemouth bass, grabbing him by the lip and lifting him out the water, feeling thoroughly proud of myself.

In the nearly three decades since, in my work as a psychologist, I've learned that therapy is a lot like fishing—if you choose the right approach for the condition you're addressing, from the dizzying array of options available, you're more likely to achieve the desired outcome. It's more complicated than I'm describing, of course, but an essential truth is this: your odds of improving are better if you rely not just on any treatment, but on treatments that work for your specific diagnosis.

In this chapter, I provide guidance and outline options for survivors of Covid-19 with mental health conditions, as well as their families, with one goal in mind: to empower them to find optimal treatment that, in my experience and that of countless patients and providers alike, helps foster thriving and not merely surviving.

ANNA'S STORY

Thirty-two-year-old Anna, a mother of three, is dynamic, effervescent, and loves many different hobbies, especially hiking. Recently, however, her light has dimmed, her enthusiasm replaced by fear. On a recent family visit to a local waterfall, a gentle walk through peaceful woodland, she suddenly fell to the ground, sweating, struggling for breath, her heart racing. After a few minutes, the feelings passed but, shaky and exhausted, she needed to head back to the car. "I'm okay," she told her wide-eyed children, but she knew she wasn't. It was the fourth panic attack she had experienced in the last couple of weeks and a sense of foreboding settled over her. She'd had a couple of similar episodes many years before, once on the evening before she boarded a plane and flew across the country to attend college in California, and again at her grandmother's funeral when she delivered a eulogy in front of hundreds of people to honor a woman who had died far too soon. But lately, after being sick with Covid, the panic attacks had been emerging frequently and for no obvious reasons at all.

During a recent visit with her general practitioner, Anna surprised herself by crying uncontrollably when her longtime provider gently asked how she was doing. After recounting her struggles with panic attacks and her constant fear of having another, she was given a referral to a therapist. Yet, a couple of weeks later, Anna has still not made an appointment. She is not convinced that talking to someone about her feelings will help her.

Anna is not alone in her reluctance to pursue treatment for a mental health condition, as research consistently shows nearly one in every two people in need never receive help.[1] Maybe you believe deep down that you could benefit from treatment or you have a referral to a mental health practitioner, yet you're finding it difficult to take the next step. Perhaps, like Anna, when you think about therapy you have an image in mind of a psychologist nodding their head over the patient lying on a couch, free-associating for hours at a time, and think such treatment couldn't possibly be useful to you. You may fear being stigmatized as weak for seeking help for emotional difficulties or you may be hoping that your problems will disappear on their own. Worries about cost and insurance benefits may be a factor in your hesitance as may concern about how much time and energy treatment will take. The idea of seeing a mental health practitioner may just seem too exhausting and overwhelming when you are dealing with the complex realities of long Covid.

However, the good news is that treatments of various kinds have been proven to be highly effective and often even transformative: they are broadly available, including during evenings and weekends, especially with the growth of telemedicine, they are often eligible for insurance reimbursement, and they don't take a lifetime to work. Chinese philosopher Lao Tzu said, "The journey of a thousand miles starts with a single step," and making an initial appointment with a mental health professional to address your challenges may be life-changing.

In the early days of my struggle with OCD, I was reluctant to admit to anyone, including myself, that I was suffering from symptoms of what was likely a mental health condition. I told myself that I was just a little anxious. That made it seem more like I might be able to handle it on my own and that I wasn't suffering from a mental illness—which I really didn't want. I was supposed to treat those with mental health conditions, not have my own. My reluctance, indeed, my resistance, to honestly own my mental health challenges lasted a couple of months, and it didn't help me in any way. When I finally decided to address the issue and set up an appointment with a therapist, I felt a mixture of relief, trepidation, and anticipation. I felt as if I might be able to find a path forward.

THE FIRST VISIT

When it was time for me to see my new mental health professional, I had first-session jitters, as have many of the people I've referred to psychologists, counselors, and psychiatrists during my career. Often, these patients ask me a few uncomfortable questions, sometimes made in jest ("Are they going to think I'm crazy?" "Will they commit me?" "What if they make me talk about my mother?"), and sometimes they have serious concerns about what the potentially frightening process might entail. I've found that taking a few minutes to help them understand what to expect can help demystify the first appointment and smooth out ongoing proceedings. Here I provide some insight into an initial visit to a therapist, usually referred to as an intake appointment.

Try to speak to the therapist before making an appointment. Most mental health professionals are available for a short conversation before the first appointment is set up to clarify details that may be important to you. Come up with a list of questions before this call while knowing that it will be a fairly brief discussion. You may have questions about the availability of in-person or telehealth sessions, insurance options, the kinds of therapy offered, diagnoses treated, the length of a session (usually forty-five to sixty minutes), a typical timeline for treatment, or their understanding of long Covid and experience with long Covid patients.

There will be paperwork to fill out. Most therapists hand you a clipboard filled with paperwork or, especially if you're meeting virtually, direct you to complete documents online. Some can be filled out ahead of the first appointment while others are best completed with the therapist present. Forms often describe the terms of engagement, policies and procedures, costs of therapy, guidelines for communication between sessions, cancellation policies, etc. Crucially, they describe therapist–client confidentiality, explaining that your privacy is a bedrock of the relationship so that you can feel safe in discussing personal and potentially difficult issues with them. They also include the limits of confidentiality and outline situations in which mental health professionals are legally required to violate confidentiality: if they learn that you are a danger to yourself or others, for example, or if they hear about incidents that may involve child abuse or elder abuse. In addition, frequently there are self-report questionnaires related to anxiety, depression, trauma, and substance use. Be sure to fill these out honestly so that your mental health professional can get a clear sense of your symptoms and struggles.

Your therapist will have many questions for you. Ideally you will have spoken to your therapist prior to making an appointment, but there is much more that they will want to know, and their questions may include:

- Tell me a little bit about your history.
- Why have you decided to seek therapy?
- What symptoms are you experiencing and how is your life affected?
- What are you expecting?
- What are your goals?
- Have you had mental health treatment before?
- Have you thought about harming yourself or others? (Don't get ruffled by this question or take it too personally as it is a standard query among mental health providers.)

These questions vary widely but they represent the beginning of a conversation that may continue for weeks, months, and, in some cases, years.

You will have questions for your therapist. By the time you meet your therapist, whether in person or via telehealth, you'll likely have already learned about them from their website or from the person who referred you. You may also have had a short phone conversation with them. During your initial visit you can expand your knowledge by asking a few simple questions, and it is a good idea to prepare them before your appointment.

- How often do you typically meet with your patients?
- What is the process of therapy like — do you set goals for me, or do we develop them together?
- Will there be homework?
- How will I know when I'm making progress and when should I expect to see some?
- What kind of outcomes do your patients usually achieve?
- Do you have a psychiatrist you can refer me to if you think I need medication?
- Can I contact you for coaching between visits?

You won't necessarily feel like much "therapy" has occurred. While patients often feel great relief that they've found a therapist, they're often surprised to learn that in the first session, relatively little "therapy" occurs. It can feel more like a getting acquainted session, a setting of expectations, and this is important for the work together that lies ahead. Problems won't be solved on day one, or depression lifted, or anxiety quelled. Try to trust the process and stay the course now that you've taken this important first action.

You and your therapist may realize that you're not right for each other and, if so, that's okay. Good therapy occurs when a strong connection, often called a fit, exists between you and your therapist. Sometimes it may hinge on deeply personal preferences, such as preferring to see a therapist of a certain gender or with a faith-based orientation, or on your need to have flexibility around telehealth options because your car is unreliable. In such cases, you would want to know before your first meeting. In other cases, a lack of connection can come down to personality clashes or differing expectations. The first session is likely too early to gauge fit and I would suggest trying a few sessions before making a change. But if you find you are truly not feeling a connection it's important to let your therapist know. A good therapist will be comfortable having this conversation with you and will work with you to help you find other resources. Equally, if your therapist believes that a different practitioner would benefit you more, perhaps based on your diagnosis, they will let you know. It's important that you don't try to force a connection, as it rarely works.

CONTINUING THE PROCESS

As you work with your therapist, treatment plans will be developed, feelings of safety and trust will increase, new patterns start to unfold, and a sense of optimism can begin to bloom. Hopefully, you'll discover the value of time and space set aside just for you with a supportive and nonjudgmental professional and that you feel cared for and validated. I find that this is especially important for people with long Covid as many report feeling dismissed and ignored on their medical journey and having someone "on your side" is empowering. That said, you'll probably find that your therapist expects you to work hard in your sessions in order to make progress, that sometimes you'll feel vulnerable and emotionally exhausted, and that it may seem as if you're regressing for a time. This is all part of the process—though always be sure to communicate your concerns and doubts, if present, to your therapist.

A key step in working together is arriving at a diagnosis in order for your mental health professional to provide the most appropriate and effective care. If you've ever been diagnosed with a condition, you could share that information but it is still important to assess your current symptoms. Figuring out which mental health condition is affecting you (or conditions if more than one) is a primary focus in early sessions—and may be revisited over time.

Every day I try to emphasize to my patients that they are far more than a diagnosis, as do many other mental health practitioners, as we are aware of the ways in which psychiatric diagnoses are used to belittle, shame, and stigmatize. However, diagnoses are important as they help inform treatment strategies and, as a practical matter, are required for health insurance coverage. A diagnosis is usually reached over several sessions based on information gleaned from direct interaction with you, from documentation provided (with your permission) by other healthcare providers, from testing (such as brief self-report tools or more comprehensive evaluations of anxiety, depression, or personality styles), and perhaps from input provided (again with permission) by your family members. In some instances, this process is straightforward, and in other cases, it can be more complicated—e.g., when someone develops changes in their motivation, mood, and behavior and it is unclear whether this is due to depression or to the development of cognitive impairment.

In the following pages, I explore treatment options for the primary mental health conditions that we commonly see in people with long Covid. You'll see that in many cases there are several different therapies available, that certain therapies are particularly effective with certain conditions, and that treatment sometimes involves a combination of both psychological and pharmacological approaches. I believe it's helpful for you and family members to have as much information as possible, to be aware that there is much more to therapy than sitting on a couch and talking to your provider about your day, that many kinds of support are available, and that you don't have to settle for treatments that don't work.

POST-TRAUMATIC STRESS DISORDER

Psychologists often have patients they can never forget, and my guess is that thirty years from now, I'll recall Rasheeda, a woman whose story powerfully shaped my understanding of medical PTSD (trauma caused by a medical incident) long before the emergence of the pandemic, and which has contributed since to my care for long haulers. In recent years I've returned to her experience again and again, so visceral, tragic, and raw, as I've thought of the ways that Covid-19 has fostered patterns of avoidance that all too often morph into PTSD and leave disrupted lives and livelihoods in their wake.

When Rasheeda was in her mid-fifties, she had successful surgery for a bowel obstruction and was looking forward to heading home after a short hospital stay. However, a couple of days later, before she could be discharged, she started experiencing intense pain in her abdomen and developed a dangerously high fever. After a radiographic procedure, she was rushed back to the operating room where a surgical towel was removed from her abdominal cavity.

This sudden and terrifying experience was profoundly traumatizing for Rasheeda and her family, and by the time I saw her for a diagnostic evaluation a few years later, she had sworn off all surgery. I learned that a bunion on her foot was causing havoc in her life, making it difficult for her to walk or to perform her job properly, and though the solution was a simple outpatient procedure, Rasheeda couldn't bring herself to go ahead with it. The very thought of surgery terrified her, sending her into a cold sweat and causing endless sleepless nights. She told me she would never agree to it in a million years. Later I learned that this dear woman had lost her job due to her inability to walk and now spent much of her time in pain and in a wheelchair.

I've seen similar stories of avoidance in many long Covid patients of mine, including Kamisha, who has now stopped going to the doctor because she is overcome with incapacitating panic anytime she has to do anything connected with her health, and Claude, who recently woke up in a hotel room while on a well-earned vacation and, feeling disoriented, thought he was back in the ICU where he had spent seventy days on a ventilator. Overcome with feelings of panic and terror that made it difficult for him to stay in the room, he cut the vacation short and, since then, has been reluctant to travel.

There are many approaches to the treatment of PTSD but the options that are most effective, widely used, and consistently recommended by academic and clinical societies are cognitive processing therapy, prolonged exposure, and eye movement desensitization and reprocessing.

Cognitive Processing Therapy (CPT)

This highly structured short-term therapy (usually made up of around twelve individual sessions with a therapist trained in the specialty) helps people to think differently about the trauma they experienced and to correct any distorted thoughts that have emerged since their exposure to it.

For patients with PTSD, CPT starts with education about the way their disorder impacts thoughts and emotions and then transitions to a series of sessions in which patients begin processing their trauma while learning how to modify their maladaptive thought patterns. Often, they use techniques such as writing about trauma and utilizing worksheets that encourage the development of skills like cognitive flexibility and reappraisal.

This therapy has proven helpful to Reggie, a patient I've seen at the ICU Recovery Center, who blames himself for contracting Covid during an impulsive visit to a barber shop. His Covid infection led to an eight-week ICU stay and now Reggie often berates himself aggressively for a "stupid decision made by a stupid man." He is learning to identify patterns of problematic thinking that have emerged in the context of his PTSD, including jumping to conclusions (such as believing that his decision to visit the barber shop precludes him from deserving a full recovery), exaggerating and minimizing (overlooking his long history of being extremely careful during the pandemic), and emotional reasoning (concluding that because he *feels* guilty, he must *be* guilty). Once Reggie, and patients like him, learn how to use these skills in therapy sessions, they start to transfer this new way of thinking to situations in the world beyond, especially in areas that involve esteem, intimacy, power or control, safety, and trust. Ultimately, they can begin to change and transform their cognitive distortions about themselves and the world. For Reggie, this means viewing himself more positively and less critically and treating himself with kindness, compassion, and grace.

Prolonged Exposure

This treatment approach enables patients to gradually face trauma-related emotions, memories, and experiences and usually consists of nine to twelve individual sessions that focus on two primary components—imaginal exposure (discussing the trauma events) during therapy sessions and in vivo exposure outside of therapy (confronting fears in real life). Breathing techniques and education about PTSD are also key components of treatment.

In imaginal exposure, patients process their trauma with their therapist by repeatedly discussing, describing, and recounting their experiences in order to unpair the trauma triggers from the emotional reactions to them. In in vivo exposure, patients intentionally confront trauma-related activities, situations, and places that may induce feelings of anxiety and fear in doses that can be tolerated—while learning that these situations are not dangerous in and of themselves. For some Covid survivors, in vivo exposure may involve watching stories about Covid-19 on the news, while others may drive by the hospital where they were admitted or visit the ICU room where they spent time on a ventilator, or those with milder illness who were never hospitalized might unwrap a Covid test kit or walk into the drug store clinic where they received a positive test result. These exposures are tailored to the needs of individual patients, and what might be appropriate for one may not be ideal for another.

Effective exposures, whether in vivo or imaginal, may create a mild degree of discomfort for patients but should not be too difficult as the idea is to gradually build up to increasingly more challenging exposures. Over time, in vivo exposure leads to desensitization or habituation, which gives patients more confidence and mastery. When people with PTSD practice avoidance so as not to relive past traumas, their fears can often become worse over time. In contrast, when they are able to lean into the things they've long avoided—as they successfully keep doctors' appointments instead of canceling them, or manage to be present at the hospital for the birth of their grandchild instead of waiting at home, or as they learn to relax even when exposed to activities that could potentially be triggering—they begin to see that the memories they've recoiled from are not dangerous to them, and gradually they can begin to live life more fully.

Eye Movement Desensitization and Reprocessing (EMDR)

This widely used approach in the treatment of PTSD was developed in the late 1980s by psychologist Dr. Francine Shapiro, who realized, while walking in the park, that her eye movements seemed to reduce the negative emotions she experienced in response to distressing thoughts.[2] She wondered if moving her eyes had caused a desensitizing effect, and this insight led to further study, clinical trials, and the development of an entire treatment methodology.

EMDR relies on what is known as an adaptive information processing model that suggests that PTSD results from inadequate processing of disturbing memories. These memories, along with the negative thoughts and emotions that existed at the time of the trauma, are often located in the body and can be reactivated. In EMDR, effective processing of these memories occurs through the use of eye movements (and other methods), which are believed to change the way that memories are stored in the brain and the body as well. This attention to the body's role in trauma is one of the unique features of EMDR.

Usually, EMDR is provided weekly or biweekly by a specially trained therapist for between six and twelve sessions, though—in some cases—people report benefiting from just a few sessions.

ANXIETY DISORDERS

Anxiety disorders are common both in the general population and in survivors of Covid, especially two specific conditions—generalized anxiety disorder and panic disorder. In countless conversations with patients, I've heard about encounters with physicians who have been brusque, patronizing, and uncaring, as they assure them that their various long Covid symptoms and problems are "just anxiety." If this has been your experience, I'm deeply sorry. Relating to patients in ways that are diminishing, perhaps even dehumanizing, is not okay, nor is it acceptable to "psychologize" real biological conditions, nor to downplay a real and life-limiting mental health condition. If you have been diagnosed with anxiety, you will know the many ways it can impact your ability to engage in life.

Studies have shown that anxiety appears to impact as many as one in three patients with long Covid.[3,4] There are numerous evidence-based approaches to treatment that experts agree are highly effective in managing anxiety disorders. These include cognitive behavioral therapy, exposure and response prevention, and mindfulness-based cognitive therapy.

Cognitive Behavioral Therapy (CBT)

CBT is based on the assumption that learned patterns of thoughts and behaviors produce and sustain emotional states—and that different and more helpful patterns can be acquired. CBT for anxiety focuses on helping patients alter their thoughts and identify and respond differently to triggers that activate new or worsening anxiety. It relies on a variety of techniques that include thought restructuring (modifying dysfunctional thinking patterns such as always assuming the worst), thought challenging (viewing thoughts from a variety of perspectives in an attempt to be objective), and relaxation training (e.g., deep-breathing exercises and meditation).

In many patients with long Covid, their anxiety often has a strong future-related orientation, meaning that they worry about whether they or their family members will contract Covid-19 again, what will happen if they do, how their children will manage if they transition to remote learning again, etc. Worries about financial security are also common as are concerns about whether they will be able to continue working or, alternatively, be eligible for disability. While these concerns may be considered common, they become "disordered" when they increase in frequency and intensity to a degree that disrupts daily functioning. Coping with uncertainty and finding ways to tolerate not knowing what the future may hold is an especially important therapeutic challenge for long haulers, and one your therapist will likely address if you experience anxiety. CBT can be effective here as it helps people recognize that many of their fears are unlikely to occur and guides them both in identifying key automatic thoughts (e.g., *I'll never get better*) that can lead to negative emotions and in developing strategies in response.

Exposure and Response Prevention (ERP)

ERP, a type of cognitive behavioral therapy that comprises modification of both thinking and behavior, involves exposing individuals to objects, situations, or thoughts that bring on anxiety in order to extinguish the underlying fear. The goal is reached by exposing people repeatedly and in increasing doses to a situation that they are avoiding; over time, as they realize that the outcome they fear hasn't occurred, their feelings of worry and avoidance decrease. ERP is particularly effective in the management of phobias (which develop in many Covid survivors) and panic disorder.

One of my long Covid patients had been especially restless while critically ill in the ICU and his healthcare team had used arm restraints. As a result, he developed severe claustrophobia, and whenever he felt trapped or shut in, he started to experience panic attacks. Riding eleva-tors was particularly difficult for him. At first, he used the stairs instead, but as his job took him to many different offices, often located in tall buildings, this wasn't a practical solution. With the help of a therapist who specialized in ERP, he was able to face his fear little by little, first stepping inside an elevator car for a few seconds but exiting before the doors closed and then, as he grew more comfortable, riding up to the second floor—first with his therapist and then by himself. Over time, he was able to ride in elevators again.

Mindfulness-Based Cognitive Therapy (MBCT)

MBCT has its roots in cognitive therapy and incorporates aspects of mindfulness (being aware of thoughts, feelings, and sensations occur-ring in the present moment), including guided meditation and breath-ing exercises, to help individuals transition away from unhelpful thought patterns that drive anxiety. This technique can be very useful when patients begin to feel overwhelmed by negative thoughts that might usually cause them to catastrophize or to become paralyzed by anxiety. Some of my long Covid patients have told me they find it help-ful to be able to pull their mind back from worries about what their future may hold and to focus on the present moment.

DEPRESSION

As described in Chapter 4, depression is extremely common in people with long Covid and can develop both as a direct result of the biological effects of Covid and due to the many stresses and circumstances that Covid can cause, such as loss of work, financial worry, upheaval in rela-tionships, and physical and cognitive disability. As with anxiety, depression can be treated with a diverse array of clinical approaches, all of which have been found to be effective in reducing symptoms and improving mood. Treatment recommendations vary widely but the following approaches have consistent scientific support:

Cognitive Behavioral Therapy for Depression (CBT-D)

When used for depression, CBT helps individuals change and modify negative and dysfunctional thought patterns that contribute to depressive symptoms. Typically delivered over twelve to twenty sessions, this active goal-directed therapy teaches techniques that may include restructuring negative thoughts and identifying cognitive distortions such as mind reading ("He thinks I'm stupid, I know it!"), all-or-nothing thinking ("She forgot my birthday, she's the worst friend ever, and I'm never going to see her again"), overgeneralizing ("My disability application was denied; I'm never ever going to get disability, no matter how many times I apply"), and personalizing ("Erin got a D on her psychology test today and is barely passing her classes — more proof that I'm a lousy mother"). Behavioral techniques are also prominent and may include relaxation and stress-reduction techniques, and giving rewards for making changes or meeting goals.

Recently a patient of mine, who struggles with depression and has been significantly debilitated by the physical effects of long Covid, told me she had gone roller-skating the week before and had enjoyed this favorite activity for more than forty minutes. I was thrilled for her as it reflected a decision on her part to leave the house, highlighted the fact that she was developing a desire to pursue pleasurable activities again, and suggested that her fatigue, long so profound, was improving. But instead of viewing this seminal event as a marker of meaningful progress, my patient shrugged it off as if it meant nothing, engaging in a common cognitive distortion known as minimizing. As we spoke more, we were able to frame her outing rather differently and she began to take great pride in her accomplishment, one that she might be able to build on for future actions.

Acceptance and Commitment Therapy for Depression (ACT-D)

ACT focuses on helping people change their relationships with their negative and unpleasant thoughts instead of trying to change those thoughts, while helping them realize they can live rich and satisfying lives even amid struggles of various kinds. This approach has been shown to be extremely effective for the treatment of a wide array of physical and mental health conditions, including depression. I have found this therapy especially helpful in my care of long Covid patients (those with and without depression), and I expand on it further in Chapter 6.

Behavioral Activation

Behavioral activation — often considered a part of a broader CBT strategy but sometimes used by itself — is an approach to the treatment of depression that uses behaviors to influence someone's mood. Research has shown that a consistent feature of people with depression is that they lose interest in activities that were once a source of meaning and pleasure and that, as they cease to engage in these, they lose the opportunity to make social connections, while losing key sources of self-esteem. In this practical approach, which is typically delivered over twelve to sixteen sessions, individuals identify previously pleasurable behaviors and engage in these in an effort to activate positive emotions. At the same time, they identify behaviors that are unhelpful and replace them with behaviors that bring pleasure. Behavioral activation relies on a variety of techniques, including monitoring the relationships between activities and mood to identify patterns (e.g., activities that make you feel good and activities that make you feel bad) that you can increase or decrease, identifying important values as a way of engaging in valued activities, and learning to be resilient and engage in activities even if you don't feel like it, as such behavior has been shown to consistently improve depression.

Psychodynamic Therapy

Psychodynamic therapy is an approach to mental health treatment that aims to help people better understand their emotions and mental processes. With its focus on developing awareness of patterns of behavior and the way they have been influenced by early life histories and experiences, it is related to psychoanalytic theory (developed by Sigmund Freud) but is far less intensive. As an understanding of the role of unresolved conflicts and feelings grows, patients learn to deal with current behaviors and issues more effectively, and their symptoms improve. Patients are seen weekly, usually for up to sixteen sessions or so when applying the short-term model that is especially effective for depression. They are encouraged to talk about their thoughts and feelings, and, over time, key topics emerge, including those that unfold between a patient and their therapist. These themes are thought to be present in other relationships as well and working through them together helps patients connect more effectively with others.

Take a patient I'll call Rachel. Rachel was raised in a chaotic household in which her mother often withdrew from life at stressful moments, leaving Rachel and her siblings at home alone for days at a time. As an adult, in her own therapy, Rachel realized that she, too, tended to hide from life at key moments. After developing exhaustion and long-term breathing issues after a Covid infection, she displayed a pattern of hopelessness and disengagement from life, believing she didn't have the ability to tackle challenges and often experiencing seasons of depression. In psychodynamic therapy, she developed new insights into the way her view of herself was powerfully influenced by her early childhood experiences. By learning new patterns of behavior in the context of her relationship with her therapist, she was able to begin a more hopeful and proactive way of relating to others. This contributed to better functionality in other areas of her life.

While individuals often experience improvements in depression during psychodynamic therapy, this method frequently appeals to those interested in gaining self-awareness and modifying aspects of their personality as opposed to targeting specific problems with mood.

Device-Based Treatments

When therapy and medication have not worked to ease depression over time, other treatments are available that may be effective, usually administered in consultation with a psychiatrist. These include transcranial magnetic stimulation (a noninvasive procedure that uses magnetic fields to stimulate nerve cells in the brain), electroconvulsive therapy (ECT, a medical procedure in which a mild electric current is passed through the brain, causing a short seizure), and deep brain stimulation (in which a doctor implants minuscule electrodes in the part of the brain that regulates mood). These are not first-line treatments for depression but I mention them here so you can talk about them with your mental health practitioner if you are interested in finding out more.

I have had just one long Covid patient who has undergone one of these less conventional treatments, in this case ECT. She was referred to a large academic center near her home in Florida after medication and therapy proved ineffective in treating her depression. In a poignant moment, her husband told me, "She's not back to herself yet but yesterday she laughed for the first time in nine months." Treatment has been arduous and, at times, difficult to tolerate but ultimately appears to be contributing to sustained improvement for her. If traditional therapies aren't working, always feel free to talk to your therapist about other options and keep an open mind about the possibility that such treatments might be appropriate, even if they may be viewed negatively in popular culture.

SUICIDALITY

As I described in Chapter 4, suicidal ideation, or having suicidal thoughts, is common in Covid survivors, as it can be a symptom of some mental health conditions such as major depression. (In some instances, it can occur in response to difficult or traumatic events when a mental health disorder is not present.) Whether active (forming or having a plan in place for ending one's life) or passive (having fleeting thoughts about not wanting to be alive), it is a concern and one that your mental health provider will likely ask about, especially if your symptoms include feelings of hopelessness and despair, often key predictors of suicide. If your therapist is concerned about the possibility that you may harm yourself, they'll share this with you and may ask you about it in a variety of ways—sometimes using very general questions and sometimes using formal tools such as the Columbia Suicide Severity Rating Scale, a short questionnaire designed to evaluate risk.

When asked about suicide, you should answer questions honestly. Many patients are concerned that a simple acknowledgment of thoughts of suicide will immediately trigger a massive and uncomfortable response, perhaps resulting in the police showing up at the door with handcuffs ready. This isn't the case. Experienced mental health professionals will not overreact to such information and will work collaboratively with you to develop plans and strategies to ensure your safety.

Over the years, like many of my colleagues, I've had many patients report suicidal ideation. While it is always a concern, it can be navigated thoughtfully and in ways that result in patients feeling less out of control. For many years, patients who were viewed as being at risk for suicide were given a "contract for safety"—an agreement, signed by both therapist and patient, in which the patient agrees not to end their life. Recent research has shown that such contracts are not always effective (one study found that among people who took their life, 65 percent had signed such a contract) and sometimes even counterproductive.[5] Current treatment approaches utilize a "safety plan" instead. Unlike contracts for safety, these focus on ways that patients can take responsibility for their safety, and are developed in a collaborative fashion, often early in the process of treatment. Components of safety plans include teaching patients to identify triggers and situations that might worsen their suicidal ideation, providing coping skills that divert suicidal thoughts (such as distractions, relaxation, and exercise), empowering patients to identify reliable sources of support for when they may be suicidal (have contact numbers on hand for your therapist, suicide prevention hotlines, family, friends, someone in your faith community, etc.), and directing them to give medications, sharp implements, and weapons to trusted friends or family members.

Mental health providers have obligations to you—both legal and moral—that must be honored if you are actively at risk of harming yourself. They will support you in finding a high level of care right away, either by asking you to go to the emergency room or to a psychiatric hospital or by accompanying you there themselves.

OBSESSIVE-COMPULSIVE DISORDER

OCD in survivors of Covid has received significantly less attention than other mental health conditions such as anxiety, depression, and PTSD, but it has proven to be a substantial problem for many. While it has historically impacted just 3 percent of the US population, OCD is estimated to impact up to 20 percent of those with long Covid, and since the beginning of the pandemic it has risen to 15 percent of people in the general population. As noted in Chapter 4, symptoms can manifest in obsessions and compulsions that cause distress and disruption in daily living.

The most effective treatment for OCD is:

Exposure Response Prevention (ERP)

OCD often improves substantially and can even go into remission *if* treated with exposure response prevention—the "gold standard" treatment. It improves little, if at all, with more conventional psychotherapies, which can lead the patient to experience great shame by encouraging them to see their intrusive thoughts as reflective of deep-seated inner conflicts. ERP, as previously described as a treatment for anxiety disorders, is a type of cognitive behavioral therapy that exposes patients to the objects, situations, or thoughts that terrify them the most and, with OCD, helps them resist the urge to engage in compulsive rituals associated with obsessions. Simply stated, as patients sit with their fears, they realize they can tolerate them without the need to engage in compulsions and, eventually, the fears lose their power.

While it is *a* treatment for anxiety, it is largely considered *the* treatment for OCD.

At the risk of sounding dramatic, I think ERP (along with Acceptance and Commitment Therapy, described in Chapter 6) saved my life, and if you're wrestling with OCD, you may find a lifeline in these approaches, too. In the months after developing OCD, I had almost constant violent, intrusive thoughts, many of which involved thoughts of stabbing myself. I wasn't suicidal and I'm not sure I was particularly depressed, but these thoughts started the moment my feet hit the floor in the morning and rarely left until I fell into bed at night, terrified, exhausted, and overwhelmed by dread that tomorrow would be the day I would lose control and act on my thoughts. In the fleeting moments when they subsided, I tried to avoid any triggers that could reactivate them, steering clear of television shows that might contain violent images, turning off the news, and staying away from the kitchen, where a set of sharp and shiny knives threatened to catch my eye.

It was during this season that my psychologist introduced me to ERP and invited me to engage in a series of tasks so terrifying that they stopped me in my tracks and regularly brought me to tears. My instinct was to hide our set of knives—put them in the cupboard or, better yet, bury them in the backyard—but she wanted me to look at them, touch them, and even hold them. The pandemic was in full swing by then and every day, as I sat at my desk in my home office, I placed a large knife next to me. At first, I did it with clenched teeth and a grimace, placing it just out of reach, utterly frightened by the thought that I was going to grab it and slash my throat or thrust it into my arm or my stomach. Gradually, over several days, which felt surprisingly quick, the presence of the knife started to induce a little less fear in me, and after a week or two I was able to grip it for a few seconds, then for a minute, then longer, until eventually I could hold the side of the knife blade against my forearm and, in time, learned not to notice the knife at all. It was the hardest thing I've ever done. Even now I'm feeling significant anxiety as I revisit a hard chapter in my life that I don't dust off very often. Over time, this process, repeated hundreds if not thousands of times, allowed me to become desensitized to intrusive thoughts by sitting with them and not responding with a compulsion, which might have included ruminating or trying to seek reassurance from my wife.

For people with long Covid, ERP often can be extremely helpful in overcoming fear of contamination (as previously mentioned, consistently identified as the most common type of OCD obsession during the pandemic) or of contracting Covid-19 again. Interventions may include moving groceries into the house and putting them away without wearing gloves, running your bare hands over the shoes you recently wore to a doctor's appointment at a hospital clinic, for three minutes a day for seven days, walking outside in the neighborhood along an empty sidewalk without wearing a mask, or walking into a crowded grocery store while wearing a well-fitting mask. These interventions and others like them, which routinely occur in the context of ERP treatment, should be done in a supervised way and only with the guidance of a trained mental health professional.

SUBSTANCE USE DISORDERS

As I discussed in Chapter 4, substance use disorders have increased during the pandemic, and experts speculate that they have accelerated in individuals with long Covid as well, although this is a question in need of further research. Substance use disorders vary widely and treatment approaches address each person's unique needs. In general, however, they can include counseling (individual, family, and group), recovery support groups such as 12-step programs, medication, intensive outpatient treatment, residential treatment, inpatient hospitalization, and detoxification—known as detox—at an inpatient medically directed program that helps individuals overcome the physiologic symptoms of withdrawal. Group therapy is the primary treatment modality and is used far more widely than individual therapy, although patients being treated for "dual diagnoses" such as substance use disorder and anxiety or depression may benefit from individual therapy as well. Often, as other mental health concerns are addressed, substance use problems can be solved more effectively.

PSYCHOSIS

As previously mentioned, while rare, psychosis has been presenting more frequently since the beginning of the pandemic, especially in those who were sick with Covid. Antipsychotic medication is often a first-line response and can be very effective. I have also found that Acceptance and Commitment Therapy (ACT, expanded upon in Chapter 6) has been valuable to a patient I recently treated. He was struggling with visual hallucinations and found them extremely distressing. Through ACT, he has come to understand that the hallucinations, while upsetting, are not the problem as much as the way that he responds to them. Using this approach, he is learning to notice them without reacting to them — even while acknowledging that this is difficult to do. We continue to work with his psychiatrist in an effort to eliminate them.

WHEN MEDICATION CAN HELP

While I've talked a lot about psychotherapies and the role that they can play in helping long haulers with mental health conditions, I would be remiss if I didn't mention psychiatric medication and even psychiatric hospitalization in recovery. In the early days of the pandemic, I worked with a patient named Maurice who had contracted Covid twice and seemed to recover well but then developed severe symptoms of anxiety, depression, and panic disorder. He worried incessantly about what might happen if he ever tested positive for Covid again. A naturally gregarious fellow, when he and his colleagues transitioned to a work-from-home situation he missed the camaraderie of the vibrant office workplace, felt intense responsibility for the welfare of the many people he was managing, and had tremendous difficulty in adjusting to the isolation of a prolonged lockdown. Both his work and his relationships with his wife and daughter started to suffer. A successful engineer, with a family he loved deeply, Maurice was highly motivated to engage in psychotherapy and was in all respects the sort of patient who typically does well in treatment—bright, insightful, nondefensive, possessing a strong support system, and deeply desiring to change. And yet despite these considerable strengths, a strong therapeutic alliance (he and I shared a close patient–therapist connection), and a thoughtful and collaborative treatment plan, he continued to struggle and some of his symptoms started to worsen over time.

Like many patients, Maurice was reluctant to take medication and yet this was a situation where I believed it could have a beneficial role to play, so I referred Maurice for a psychiatric consultation. While we were waiting for his initial appointment, new symptoms emerged, including seeing darting black images out of the corner of his eye and going days at a time without sleeping. I decided to refer Maurice for a psychiatric consultation at the emergency room, which led to a brief *voluntary* psychiatric hospitalization where medications were started, and he was monitored in a controlled setting. I've italicized the word *voluntary* because it is always ideal when patients decide to seek inpatient treatment on their own terms. The integration of psychiatric medication into his treatment led to dramatic improvement, and, over the next year, sustained progress. As Maurice's anxiety and hallucinations decreased, he was better equipped to participate in and receive benefits from therapy. Less distressed and preoccupied by his symptoms, he was able to focus on the concepts we were discussing and more able to concentrate on engaging in homework, tasks that previously were difficult, if not impossible, for him.

This story could be repeated dozens of times and it highlights the absolutely critical role that medications can and do play. I'm generally not in favor of relying on them as a first resort, particularly in cases where symptoms are mild and where psychotherapy has not yet been attempted. Prescribing medication is often done a little too casually, sometimes by well-meaning general practitioners who prescribe far more psychiatric medications than do psychiatrists (by some estimates, they prescribe up to 80 percent of antidepressants). Having said that, relying on medications only as a last resort is also unwise. In many cases, optimal mental health treatment involves the use of both psycho-therapy and medication. I have found that combining these two approaches has been helpful in my mental health journey, as well as in the journeys of many of my patients, and this may be true for you as well.

Some patients who are happy to talk to a therapist are hesitant to take medication, frequently because of stereotypes that are largely inaccurate but also culturally entrenched. In my work, the primary objections I hear are the fear that psychiatric medications are addictive (they generally aren't), that they have undesirable side effects (some-times they do, although these typically improve with time and most patients find them manageable), and that they don't work (few treat-ments work 100 percent of the time but they are usually helpful and sometimes profoundly so). As you embark on a relationship with your therapist, please feel the freedom to have a candid conversation with them about the role that pharmacologic treatment can have in your care, and consider maintaining an open mind about ways that psychiat-ric medications can improve your symptoms and your life.

ANNA'S STORY

At the beginning of the chapter, I introduced my patient Anna, who was experiencing new and frequent panic attacks but couldn't see how talking to a therapist would improve her situation. After another panic attack, this time at the grocery store, she realized that her attacks were initially driven by reading about rising Covid rates or hearing about friends, neighbors, and former classmates becoming ill from the virus, but, increasingly, they seemed to be triggered by situations that had nothing to do with Covid, such as a conversation with her husband, who shared that he was thinking about quitting his job and starting a business, or being in crowded places. Sometimes, as in the most recent one, they were triggered by nothing at all.

As soon as she made it home from the store, she called the psychologist that her doctor had referred her to, a specialist in the management of anxiety-related conditions, including panic attacks. "I don't think it will make things worse," she told her husband that evening over dinner, "and, you never know, maybe it will help." After an initial phone conversation with the therapist, Anna set up an appointment for the next week and then began a course of therapy sessions that combined elements of cognitive behavioral therapy and ERP. She was surprised by the hands-on, practical components of each and found that, over time, the strategies she learned helped decrease her anxiety in a variety of situations. In particular, she was glad to have tools at the ready when needing to navigate crowds and during the planning of a visit to see her mother in Puerto Rico, where she worried that she and her family might get stranded if another lockdown happened. Within months, her panic attacks had decreased considerably as she had a new understanding of the stresses that activated her feelings of intense anxiety, and while her underlying anxiety hadn't completely disappeared, she had learned methods to manage it more effectively. When it was time to go on their long-planned trip, she didn't cancel it as she thought she might, but rather she managed to have—with periodic difficulty—an "amazing time." Her story is not an unusual one and can be the story of millions of long haulers if they have access to appropriate resources.

I've always loved the poem "The Road Not Taken" by Robert Frost, a moving reflection on the critical importance of choices. It has especially resonated during these difficult pandemic years. We all grapple with decisions, and it seems apt to think of the poem in the context of choosing how to proceed with mental health care, particularly the final stanza, in which the narrator notes, "Two roads diverged in a wood, and I—/ I took the one less traveled by, / And that has made all the difference." As I've reflected on my struggle with OCD, I've often thought about this idea, of standing at a fork in a road in the fall of 2018 when my symptoms first showed their fangs and having two distinct options: to pursue mental health treatment or grit my teeth, hide my story, and try to go it alone. At the time, the first option seemed the hardest by far, but sitting here today, I can hardly believe that I leaned strongly toward the second possibility, but I did. I remember wistfully thinking that my obsessive thoughts might magically disappear as quickly as they came, that they might vanish if I changed my diet a bit, that I could pray them into oblivion, and that, if these strategies failed, I could always keep a stiff upper lip and soldier on. I'm hoping that if you were in a similar situation at the beginning of the chapter, desperately avoiding acknowledging that you have a mental health condition and studiously sidestepping treatment for it, you now might have changed your mind. That you might decide to take that first step, that road less traveled, to getting the support and effective treatment you need now that you've seen the multiple available options and pathways toward healing.

I hope so.

CHAPTER 6

REFRAMING YOUR NEW NORMAL:
The Role of Acceptance as a Pathway to Healing

Ronnie is a Covid survivor and one of the more remarkable people I know. Having spent forty-nine days desperately ill on a ventilator, he's a little shocked and surprised at times that he's alive, and while grateful, sometimes he's deeply sad as he contemplates the ways both large and small that his illness has upended his life.

A middle-aged teacher from a Southern town, he is on a leave of absence from work and passes his time at home, his anxiety never far away and his symptoms of PTSD often nipping at his heels. But perhaps the most constant feature of his new existence is a portable oxygen tank, a tip of the cap, sadly, to lungs that were badly damaged by Covid pneumonia and that, two years later, have not fully recovered, leaving him easily fatigued. Oxygen tanks can be a lot like Rorschach ink blots—they trigger reactions in people—and, for a long time, Ronnie's tank symbolized for him everything that had gone wrong in his life, a dream-filled future permanently stunted, adventures cut short, and family memories never realized. But, over the past few months, he started to have a change of heart.

Bolstered by insights from Acceptance and Commitment Therapy, he began to understand that he could accomplish hard things even with damaged lungs and while struggling with his mental health. The idea of taking his first vacation since leaving the hospital started to form in his mind and he hatched a plan for a family visit to a Minor League Baseball park one state away. I enthusiastically endorsed the trip—it wouldn't be easy nor absurdly hard but perhaps just right. At first, when Ronnie filled me in on details, his voice was wistful as he talked about the many excursions he and his family had once taken, describing far-flung cities visited and items on bucket lists checked off. A trip to a tiny Double-A stadium on the edge of a cornfield next to a Walmart would never have been his idea of an adventure and yet, here we were, push-ing the envelope of what he believed was possible and wrestling with the idea that he could make space for a new normal in his life.

As the day of the baseball pilgrimage drew close, his excitement grew. During our sessions, he worried whether his oxygen tank could run out, what would happen if he fell ill while driving through one of dozens of small rural towns, whether he would have the stamina to walk to his seat in the outfield. But he didn't think of canceling. He was determined to make the expedition work. He had come to see that driving a few hundred miles to watch the Biloxi Shuckers play the Montgomery Biscuits might not be the same as flying to Los Angeles to watch the Dodgers against the Padres—but it could be part of a new and satisfying life.

ACTION AND COMMITMENT THERAPY (ACT)

In this chapter, I'll explore Acceptance and Commitment Therapy, an innovative approach to therapy shown to be effective with patients expe-riencing chronic illness, including people like Ronnie living with long Covid. Over the past few years, I've often reached out to my psychology colleagues, seeking and sharing advice, and widening my knowledge in my endeavor to best treat my patients. In the informal surveys I've con-ducted, I've found they regularly report ACT (pronounced *act*) as one of their treatments of choice for long haulers. It is not designed to target any specific form of mental illness but rather to empower people to create rich and meaningful lives, even while acknowledging the pain and frustration of current struggles—and accepting their accompanying thoughts and feelings. ·

Developed in 1984 by psychologist Steven C. Hayes, a professor at the University of Nevada, ACT is part of the broad family of cognitive and behavioral therapies and is generally regarded as one of the third-wave behavioral therapies—clinical approaches that sit outside of those historically practiced in the West and that highlight the importance of concepts such as acceptance, self-compassion, and mindfulness rather than placing an emphasis on the reduction or elimination of psychological and emotional symptoms—although that is often the outcome. While many other therapeutic strategies are based on "healthy normality," the idea that humans are naturally psychologically healthy and that psychological suffering is abnormal—a disease that needs to be reduced or eliminated—ACT embraces the idea that so-called negative human emotions are part of human experience and focuses not on their eradication but on a person's relationship to them. Based on empirical data, ACT has been found to be effective in the treatment of substance use disorder,[1] psychosis,[2] anxiety,[3] depression,[4] chronic pain,[5] and eating disorders.[6] In my care of patients living with long Covid, like Ronnie, I've learned how ACT offers hope for them and their families as they encounter new and unwanted challenges, wrestle with unpleasant thoughts and situations, and try to stay true to who they are in the process.

Ronnie's story is deeply personal to me as I care about him, but also because, in many ways, his story parallels my own. I wasn't in the ICU with Covid, but my OCD is an oxygen tank of sorts, and for a long time I thought its very presence would limit me and prevent my happiness and flourishing. And like Ronnie, who scoffed at the idea of thriving with a damaged set of lungs, anxiety, and PTSD, I couldn't imagine how I could coexist, much less excel, with a mental illness. Shortly after my diagnosis, I told my psychologist, with all the authority I could muster, that other people might be willing to live with a chronic mental health condition but not me. I was insulted that she even wanted me to consider such a thing. I was a scrappy underdog from a small town who overcame challenges, a grizzled former college wrestler who imposed his will on things, a resourceful medical school professor who was skilled at finding answers if they existed, and I was determined to view OCD as just a problem to solve, not an illness to accept.

I spent hundreds of hours scouring the internet looking for a cure, emailing researchers conducting clinicals trials on nutrition and OCD so frequently that I worried that it might look like I was stalking them, and trying to convince myself that if I got a little more sleep and dramatically reduced my stress, my mental illness would go away. It was only later that I realized, with my therapist's help, that while it felt as if I were working hard, my actions were actually a form of avoidance — and they were creating an additional layer of problems for me. Luckily for me, my therapist introduced ACT into my treatment, and when I started to embrace the truth about my illness, instead of running from it, my life started to change.

SIX PILLARS OF ACT

The ultimate goal of ACT is to develop increased psychological flexibility, defined by Hayes as "making contact with experience in the present moment fully and without defense," and its key tenets help people move toward it. ACT's six pillars are:

Acceptance

Also referred to as *expansion,* acceptance is the process of making room for upsetting and distressing thoughts, feelings, attitudes, and experiences instead of resisting, denying, and defending against them. In

ACT terminology, acceptance is expressed through the "Four *A*s" — acknowledge, allow, accommodate, and appreciate.

- *Acknowledge* is to recognize and notice the presence of thoughts and feelings.
- *Allow* is deciding to let them exist and choosing not to push them away.
- *Accommodate* is the willingness to make room for them, whatever they might be.
- *Appreciate* is to not necessarily like them but to reflect on them and recognize that even unpleasant thoughts and emotions can be beneficial and helpful.

When talking with my long Covid patients about the concept of acceptance, whether in connection with the new reality of their lives or the waves of emotion that they may be feeling, I use the analogy of an unwanted houseguest to bring the Four *A*s to life. It often helps them grasp the idea as they think of the journey from fighting with or actively avoiding the guest to appreciating that their presence may be beneficial. You might find it helpful, too, in starting to apply the Four *A*s in your own life.

Peter, a middle-aged emergency room nurse, had a mild case of Covid-19 that led him to develop significant cognitive problems that made it difficult to carry out his demanding job. Currently, he's on a temporary disability leave, which has left him feeling depleted and depressed, but until recently, he's been reluctant to acknowledge his sadness about having long Covid. Instead, he has soothed and distracted himself with food and endless escapes into movies or television shows whenever he's feeling down. He has felt misunderstood by his friends and spends a lot of time alone, telling everyone that he is "just fine."

I've been working with Peter for some months now and introduced key concepts from ACT. Over time, he has begun to notice his sadness and instead of pushing it away and retreating, he tries to embrace his emotions whenever they emerge, allowing them to wash over him. He is beginning to feel less defensive and is learning that these painful feelings often diminish rather than worsen if he is willing to sit with them and experience them, instead of running away or, worse yet, trying to lock them deep inside. With the acceptance of his sad feelings, he is in a better place to be able to manage them, and now, some nights, instead of watching hour upon hour of TV, he plays his guitar again, a sure way, he's found, to lift his spirits. He's starting to think about reaching out to one of his old work buddies to get together and play some music, just like they used to do.

Another patient, Cara, is an aspiring singer-songwriter in her twenties who was hospitalized with Covid-19. With damaged lungs due to the effects of her illness, her voice sounds different from the way it did before, and she has been reluctant to sing at venues, convinced that she'll be booed off stage. For months, Cara turned down potential gigs, hoping that her old voice would magically reappear, feeling angry and frustrated in the meantime. Over time, she began to try to accept that her new voice was here to stay and that any hope of a singing career was over, and she channeled her emotions into new songs—that maybe other people would sing. As she did so, she surprised herself by wondering what would happen if she continued to sing herself. What if people didn't mind the new voice?

Recently, during our weekly session, she shared with me that she had summoned the courage to go on stage at an open mic night the evening before. "And guess what?" she said. "People loved my raspy voice! And the songs." One person in the audience had compared her to the singer Stevie Nicks—which Cara took as a huge compliment. While she still doesn't love her voice, she's beginning to acknowledge it as part of her story—and to see how the person she is now is reflected in the soulful songs she has started to write, resonant with a full range of human emotions, and so different from her previous repertoire of cheerful pop songs.

Strategies for embracing acceptance include:

- Trying to be aware of the process that happens within you when uncomfortable thoughts, attitudes, feelings, and sensations arise. Do you find yourself shutting them down?
- Considering the ways that you do this. It might be through distraction or by distancing yourself. It's likely that you have a go-to method.
- Thinking of previous times when you've avoided difficult thoughts and emotions and whether it was beneficial.
- The next time you feel uncomfortable emotions, trying not to fight, or avoid, but create space for them to exist.
- Not feeling the need to fix or change anything. Letting the emotion wash over you.
- Starting small if you find this challenging. Sitting with the emotion for a short time, building up gradually.

Cognitive Defusion

Cognition defusion, also known as *thought defusion,* or simply *defusion,* is the practice of creating separation between oneself and one's thoughts and feelings—that is, developing the ability to observe thoughts and feelings without allowing them to define you, identifying too fully with them, or accepting them as the absolute truth. In many approaches to therapy, the primary goal is to change or modify thoughts but in ACT the aim is to change your relationship *with* them.

When I think of patients who have had success with cognitive defusion, my mind turns to Earl, a small business owner in his late fifties who has experienced significant disappointments in his life. Most recently he faced financial insecurity as his small Nashville restaurant failed. Once a promising and profitable business selling hot chicken, a local culinary staple, it cratered as the entire county went into lockdown during the pandemic. Not long after, Earl contracted Covid and by the time he arrived at my clinic, he was battling problems with fatigue as well as depression and cognitive dysfunction. Frustrated and discouraged by his struggles and the downward trajectory of his life, he constantly thought about himself as a failure and a disappointment. "No wonder my wife left me," he would add. It was difficult for him to see these thoughts as distorted thinking, a hallmark of major depressive disorder, as he believed the evidence that proved them right was clear to everyone. Instead, he took them on board as the absolute truth in ways that prevented him from moving forward with his life. *What's the point?* he questioned when presented with potential tools or solutions. *I'll just mess everything up. It won't work for me!* He had become completely fused with his thoughts.

For Earl, who had tried various treatments for depression, ACT has started to make a real difference. He is learning to notice his thoughts for what they are — words or images passing through his mind. When he thinks, *You're a failure*, now he is able to say to himself, "I'm having the thought that I'm a failure again." In doing so, he is more easily able to not assign any value to it and remind himself that thoughts are just thoughts, not necessarily facts. This simple technique has taken away the power his thoughts once had to define the narrative of his life.

Other cognitive defusion strategies include:

- Allowing thoughts to come and go without latching on to them. Imagining they are fish swimming in a stream or leaves floating along the surface while you watch them drifting away from you.
- Being curious and open to thoughts as they arise without reacting to them.
- Asking yourself whether these thoughts are helpful to you.
- Asking if the thoughts are true.

Contact with the Present Moment

This concept reflects ACT's emphasis on awareness of what psychologists call the here and now — being attuned to, engaged in, and focused without judgment on what is happening in the moment. It is also known as mindfulness. By living in the present, people can avoid two unproductive extremes: ruminating about past events that can't be altered and worrying about a future that may not happen and cannot be controlled. This doesn't mean that we shouldn't be thinking about the past or planning for the future, as both can be helpful and necessary. The key here is to not let today be buried under an avalanche of thoughts associated with things that have come and gone or not yet happened.

I often observe that many of my long Covid patients spend hours reflecting on the way things were prior to contracting Covid. In many cases, their lives have changed drastically, and they are no longer able to participate in countless activities they once took for granted, and I try to validate their feelings. However, if their practice of looking to the past causes them to feel increasingly sad about their current situation, it can be helpful to find ways to focus on the here and now. Similarly, many of my patients ruminate on future scenarios that may never happen, such as experiencing a significant increase in their symptoms, losing gains they have made, or perhaps developing dementia. This can lead to an acceleration of anxiety that adds to their already heavy burden. Grieving the past even while worrying about the future is a normal reaction to a major life change, but if it impacts the way you engage your current challenges or prevents you from being fully present in your life or in relationships with others, mindfulness tools can be extremely valuable. I find it resonates with my patients when I remind them that the current moment is the only place in which we have power and the possibility of making choices about our lives.

Margie is a minister at a church in a nearby community and the survivor of a forty-day hospital stay initiated by a severe case of Covid. Her quiet, ordered existence changed dramatically after her critical illness as she now finds herself navigating hospitalizations to address medical problems, frequent doctors' visits, significantly diminished cognitive abilities, and worsening anxiety. Her mind is often filled with worries about her health and questions about her future but, in the midst of all this, she is grateful to be alive. We have worked together for some months now, using the concepts of ACT, and she is beginning to fold them into her life. Every week, she gladly preaches at her church, sitting in a chair as standing is exhausting now, and somewhat less eloquently than before, her words looping and repeating due to cognitive dysfunction. Over time, she has adjusted to this new reality with patience and grace, finding it especially helpful not to dwell on the past or worry about the future but to embrace the moments when she looks out over her congregation and sees her words, especially heartfelt these days, reaching them and making a difference in their lives.

A wide array of tools and techniques is available to help people stay in the present moment, and many of my patients have found their ability to be mindful increases by slowing down and noticing their surroundings (sights, sounds, smells), practicing meditation, engaging in breathing exercises, and developing a deeper awareness of bodily sensations, senses, and emotions. I like to start by encouraging patients to practice being present while doing any and all activities, no matter how mundane (such as brushing their teeth, putting gas in the car, biting into an apple, or hammering a nail into a wall), through developing engaging, savoring, and focusing skills. You may find these helpful:

- *Engaging skills* involve turning our full attention to an activity, making sure that we are not multitasking, and pulling thoughts and focus back to the present moment if we find them drifting away to the past or future. This might include describing the activity — "I'm moving the toothbrush over my back teeth. I like the way the toothpaste smells minty and fresh."
- *Savoring skills* guide people to savor or gain pleasure from an activity — such as noticing the marvelously sweet and slightly tart taste of a single blueberry as you eat it slowly (as opposed to gobbling down handfuls at dinner, as I often do).
- *Focusing skills* involve learning to attend to the most important part of an activity, while noticing other elements as well — such as watching a bobber move from side to side on the surface of the

water while fishing, and taking in the sounds of birdsong and the movement of frogs jumping from lily pads into the pond.

Values

One of the unique features of ACT is an unabashed emphasis on values, which, traditionally, are seldom discussed in psychotherapy. According to ACT, values are principles that guide and motivate us, and give our lives meaning. They are personal and may change over time. Not to be confused with goals, which are attainable and often discarded once reached, values can provide direction in our lives. The book *ACT Made Simple* by Russ Harris sums it up well: "Values are like a compass. A compass gives you direction and keeps you on track when you're traveling. And our values do the same for the journey of life. We use them to choose the direction in which we want to move and to keep us on track as we go. So when you act on a value, it's like heading west. No matter how far west you travel, you never get there; there's always further to go."

Values may include acceptance, authenticity, belonging, courage, dignity, family, freedom, gratitude, healing, justice, kindness, love, safety, self-compassion, and many others, and can arise by questioning what is important to you in your life. You can reflect on your values by asking yourself questions: "How would I choose to have my life unfold?" or "What do I want for my life going forward?" As you identify values, it helps you to see the big picture of your life, the long term, and to begin to make choices that align with these values.

In our long Covid support groups, we often ask our patients about their values and how they may have changed during their illness. I have seen many rich and long conversations develop on this important topic. Common values endorsed by our patients include family and relationships, self-care, living without guilt, and living according to their faith. Honoring these values in the face of realities brought on by the impact of their illness has led to changes in behavior for many of them. For example, one support group member, Tara, who is challenged with overwhelming fatigue, now carefully prioritizes how she spends her time, choosing to expend energy by sitting with her daughters while they do homework, or by lying on the couch watching a movie with her husband in the evening. Almost everything else is off-limits for now. Others have learned to treat themselves with gentleness, compassion, and understanding, reflecting a dawning awareness of how precious they are.

During the early stages of my OCD journey, I participated in a support group led by a psychologist specializing in ACT, and we spent many hours reflecting on key values, talking them over, and going through worksheets with dozens of examples. The value that resonated the most with me was freedom: the ability to go where I wanted, do what I wanted, watch what I wanted, and listen to what I wanted without being afraid of the many intrusive thoughts that these activities might trigger. At the time, I was speaking regularly at academic meetings and giving lectures across the country, and I was increasingly worried that I would say something profane or sexually explicit during a presentation, so much so that I had begun to lighten my load and decrease the number of talks I was giving. Sitting with the other group members, and looking at the worksheet of values, I realized that I wanted to walk in freedom and to confidently engage in meaningful pursuits, even if doing so was distressing. This knowledge gave me the motivation to learn how to lean into my fears to continue speaking to healthcare professionals about translating insights from research into better patient care—something I love very much.

Strategies for defining your values include:

- Thinking about what you want for your life now.
- If you find yourself listing goals, trying to tease out the values at their heart.
- Considering what matters to you—what makes you happy, sad, or angry.
- Thinking about when you feel inspired.

- Considering times you have felt grateful or appreciative.
- Giving some thought to the different people and relationships in your life. Who do you want to spend time with, and how?

Committed Action

Once values have been clarified, it is possible to take the next step of moving forward with committed action—action in the direction of what is important to us, guided by our values. Not surprisingly, choosing to live by and honor our values can be challenging and often requires making difficult decisions, some of which may create discomfort. Yet value-driven action has served many of my long Covid patients well, and I've marveled as I've witnessed them engaging in hard, sometimes terrifying, actions, inspired by a desire to honor important commitments they've made to themselves or others.

Margie, a retired seamstress, has a ninety-five-year-old father as well as aunts, uncles, and cousins who live in Texas—almost a thousand miles away from her home in Tennessee. After two years of missing physical contact with them during the pandemic, *family connection* was number one on her list of values when she wrote them down during a session. Margie decided that she *must* go and see them, but the question was how, as the hurdles she needed to overcome to do so were legion. She had just turned seventy-three, had recently recovered from a broken hip, and had endured significant cognitive challenges since developing Covid—meaningful problems with her attention and memory that contributed to often getting lost while driving and to forgetting where she had put her keys, eyeglasses, and medications. She also battled striking fatigue, sometimes confined to the couch for a day or two after she pushed herself hard. The idea of taking a flight to Dallas, wandering through DFW Airport, then boarding another plane to Waco while lugging a suitcase, wearing a mask, and trying to stay six feet away from others was daunting. What if she were to get lost and miss her connecting flight? Or misplace her ticket? These thoughts filled her with fear and yet the idea of not being with her family for the second Thanksgiving in a row bothered her even more. She knew that if she wanted to see her family, she had to find a way to travel to the Lone Star State.

In an impressive feat of planning, problem-solving, creating backup plans, and managing distress tolerance, she made the trip, arriving intact even if her eyeglasses were lost somewhere en route. A few days later, when her exhaustion had lifted and she sat down with her father and other family members at a Thanksgiving table crowded with food, she knew that her trip, propelled by her values, had been more than worth the challenges she'd faced.

Traveling across the country is a bridge too far for some long haulers, including several of my patients, whose fatigue is so profound that a move from couch to chair is challenging and for whom flying for hours or, for that matter, driving to the airport is inconceivable. In these situations, committed action looks different from Margie's but can still contribute to involvement in meaningful pursuits. One of my patients has started raising chickens for their eggs since developing long Covid, and while this is enjoyable for her, it is also a reflection of one of her core values, protecting the planet via sustainability. Unrelenting fatigue—her primary symptom, though she has many—has made it difficult to engage in life with the fullness and vitality that she once did, but she is often able to bask in the sun with her partner, a floppy hat shielding her from the heat, watching her birds and knowing that she is doing her own small part to help the environment. She considers her chickens her pets and these moments, brief as they are, remain a source of great joy and meaning in her life.

Self-as-Context

Perhaps the most complicated ACT concept to describe, *self-as-context* is also referred to as the *observing self* or the *core you*, the transcendent and constant part of us that notices all our shifting internal and external experiences. It contrasts with the *conceptualized self*, the self that is defined by the content of our lives, including facts, subjective details, the roles we play, and the stories that we tell ourselves about who we are (e.g., I'm on the track team in college, I'm a parent, I like dogs, I'm a leader at work, I'm the patient one in my family, I'm a long hauler, etc.). It can be helpful to think of the observing self as not defined by these shifting roles we adopt in the world but as simply watching. One of the primary aims of ACT is to disentangle the relationship between the observing self and the conceptualized self in an effort to help people understand that they are distinct from their achievements, labels, failures, and successes, and, importantly, their medical diagnoses, and to prevent them from overidentifying with these stories and self-concepts, which are just constructions and *not* who we are.

Long Covid's impact on wide-ranging aspects of physical, mental, and cognitive health as well as areas such as family, finances, and work is so all-encompassing that many of my patients find it difficult to stop it from defining them. Just as live kudzu vines (familiar to many of us who live in the South) overtake trees, plants, fences, abandoned houses, and almost everything in their path, long Covid often wraps its tentacles around people so thoroughly that it can be the only thing they see about themselves. While this is understandable, it can be unhelpful. In such instances, guiding people to consider that there is a part of them that is distinct from being a long hauler can be beneficial.

Recently, I had a conversation with one of my support group patients about this. Jon is an admissions counselor at a local college, though he is currently on leave after a Covid infection left him with a vast array of physical symptoms (heart palpitations, dizziness, debilitating fatigue, and problems regulating temperature) that have persisted for more than two years and still show no evidence of abating. He often feels as if his home has become his personal prison as he can only rarely leave its confines and, far too often, his only daily activity is moving from the bed to the couch and back to the bed again. He sees himself now primarily through the lens of his chronic illness and everything that entails.

We continue to work with Jon—and with all our support group

members—on creating distance from his conceptualized self and on helping him become less attached to his current perception about who he is. This is no simple thing. However, I've consistently found that long haulers like Jon are open to the possibility that they are far more than the sum of their current disabilities and limitations, that they have the ability to modify the narratives they create about themselves, and that the core you, their inner self, is still there—especially when this idea is presented with empathy and an acknowledgment of the profundity of their struggles. In Jon's case, he's been able to unhook himself from his long Covid diagnosis, trying not to let it define who he is. He has allowed himself to accept that he is still a loving father to his grown-up daughter, a mentor and role model to a couple of his former students, and a patient owner of a playful cat.

Strategies for using self-as-context include:

- Thinking about the different roles you take on in the world, both consciously and unconsciously, and seeing if you can broaden your view of yourself.
- Watching, listening, and simply noticing the psychological and physical experiences of your life, and recognizing that the core you remains unchanged.

PSYCHOLOGICAL FLEXIBILITY IN ACTION

Psychological flexibility, the ultimate goal of ACT, known to many experts as the psychological superpower, encompasses the ability to cope with and adapt to difficult circumstances, be aware of the present moment, even when unpleasant thoughts and feelings arise, and behave and respond in ways that honor your values.

My patient Ronnie is a good example of someone who has developed a degree of flexibility in his responses to thoughts and emotions and has stayed committed to his values of family connection and, in his words, "seizing the day." In arranging his visit to a Minor League

Baseball game, he found a novel way to fuel his sense of adventure with his family, while dealing with the challenge of having to accept his limitations and overcoming setbacks along the way.

The day of his outing came, and with great trepidation and a touch of enthusiasm, he set off with his family, stopping at a country store or two along the way to pick up supplies. The journey was long and tiring but when he made it to his seat in the bleachers, his wife and daughter on either side, he leaned back and smiled. He wasn't thinking about journeys he had once taken or worrying about his oxygen tank. Instead, he munched on peanuts and Cracker Jack and cheered loudly for his new favorite team. His life was happening now.

One hot summer day in Portage, Michigan, in 1977, I was playing baseball with my cousin Donny. Well, not exactly baseball. We were in a weed-strewn vacant lot across the street from my house, Donny waiting a hundred feet or so away from me with his new Wilson glove while I stood at a makeshift plate, throwing a ball into the air, and hitting it as far as I could with an old wooden bat. After a few pop-ups and a line drive or two, I sent a towering fly ball over Donny's head (much higher than the glove he hurled into the air), and it landed with a sickening thud against the windshield of a brand-new truck parked beside a building that bordered the field. In my time, I've told a few lies and cheated on a Spanish test or two but not that day. There was only one thing to do—to walk to the brown cinder-block building, introduce myself to the man inside, and admit that I had broken his truck window. It was a hard thing to do and even the idea of it caused me great distress, but I did it, propelled by my values.

I've thought about this story a lot in recent years, sometimes joking about it with my cousin, but I've found it most helpful in moments of discouragement when I've doubted that I have the mettle to accept and lean into hard and unwanted things and have thought that avoidance would be a far better choice. I'll, of course, be the first to admit that my simple story pales in comparison to the difficulties that long haulers are challenged to navigate *every single day*. The hard things that *you* have in

front of you—and that I'm inviting you to make room for and accept—
are inestimably difficult. But you may find that in being open to the
ideas of ACT, it is possible to engage the present situation as it is (*not as
you want it to be*) and make space for distressing thoughts and feelings;
guided by overarching values, you can take committed action to do
difficult things and find meaning in the process.

CHAPTER 7

THE WOUND IS WHERE THE LIGHT ENTERS: Post-traumatic Growth After Covid

In his classic autobiographical work, *Man's Search for Meaning,* Austrian psychiatrist, philosopher, and author Viktor Frankl observed that individuals can endure hugely difficult things if they are able to find meaning in them and that they can even be transformed in the process. A survivor of several concentration camps during World War II, he lost his father, mother, wife, and brother to the atrocities of the Nazi regime, and his writing and philosophies grew out of personal experience. Against this stark backdrop of tragedy, he developed logotherapy, a therapeutic approach (that some describe as more of a philosophy than a therapy) based on the premise that people are primarily driven by a desire for meaning in life, and that meaning can be experienced and created, even in the midst of suffering. In *Man's Search for Meaning,* Frankl states that his theories helped him survive the inhumane treatment in the camps, and that his experience there confirmed and advanced his beliefs.

As I've worked with patients, perhaps especially during the Covid-19 pandemic, I've come to appreciate the essential truth of Frankl's insights—that when lives and livelihoods are derailed, and hopes and dreams are dashed, there is often meaning to be found that can lead to paths out of the abyss and even opportunities to flourish. Many of my patients, including those living with long Covid, have discovered that difficult endings, perhaps of the way life used to be, can give way to new and meaningful beginnings, that life transformations can occur in the midst of struggle and may even be fostered and facilitated. In this chapter, my aim is to elaborate on Frankl's key tenet—*growth can occur through facing hard things*—and introduce the concept of post-traumatic growth, a psychological change that can arise as people cope with traumatic events in their lives, including debilitating illness. You may have noticed this yourself as you've navigated the complexities of long Covid.

A few years ago, I was invited to give a keynote lecture on PTSD at a conference on humanity in ICU care at a medical center in Albuquerque, New Mexico. Standing at the podium, I talked about the paradoxes I had observed in the lives of ICU survivors I worked with, how their lives were harmed by critical illness and yet were often transformed in positive ways in the process. I had witnessed these changes unfold with enough of my patients that it had caught my attention, and humbled me, as they sought to find a new way forward in their lives. I concluded my lecture with a reference to a verse from the Old Testament Book of Isaiah that, over the years, has captured for me the extraordinary transformation that can occur amid difficult life events. It describes an exchange—"beauty for ashes"—of replacing despair with something life-fulfilling. The promise of hope from grief. The meaning transcends its religious origins.

The conference was funded by a woman named Caroline, whose husband had experienced an untimely death in the ICU, and, later that evening, I was able to meet her and have dinner with her and her family at a charming Mexican restaurant in the city's Old Town neighborhood. Just before we sat down to eat, she pulled me aside to say that on hearing the words *beauty for ashes,* she had almost fallen out of her chair.

She had embraced this phrase after her husband's death and even used it now as the first part of her email address. She told me that, in her grief, she had come to realize just how brief life was and had determined to live the remainder of her life in a purposeful and impactful way, using her resources to help support education and advocacy efforts to ensure the thoughtful care of critically ill patients, ICU survivors, and their families. "I wanted to find meaning in my husband's death," she said. "To have something good come from it."

THE CONCEPT OF POST-TRAUMATIC GROWTH

While the concept of personal transformation emerging from traumatic life events is not new, the term *post-traumatic growth* (PTG) was coined in the 1990s by Richard Tedeschi and Lawrence Calhoun, psychologists at the University of North Carolina.[1] Since then, they have pioneered research and theories in the field, and PTG is now an established concept in the world of psychology. In general, it rests on the idea that significant trauma—sometimes after a single event but sometimes, in my work experience, in the context of a struggle with ongoing events or major negative life disruptions, such as living with chronic illness—can shake up someone's life so profoundly that it can cause people to question fundamental assumptions, deeply held views about themselves, their world, and their future. Through the process of cognitive engagement, in which people reflect on the trauma they have endured and find ways to make sense of it, growth can begin to occur as core beliefs are reconsidered and challenged, old value systems dismantled, and new values, priorities, and life goals are established. While the term *post-traumatic growth* suggests that transformation occurs in the aftermath of trauma, I've noted that with the long Covid patients I care for—whose struggles are multifaceted and ongoing—it can arise concurrently as they deal with their difficult experience, perhaps as their insights grow or as small steps of progress are made.

The exact prevalence of PTG is hard to determine, and its

magnitude varies widely, but most investigations suggest it is experienced to some degree by approximately one in two people after exposure to trauma[2] (with some studies suggesting that PTG may occur in nearly 90 percent[3]), including in those with life-threatening illnesses such as cancer. Data show that it is more likely to arise in women than men[4] and in people younger than 60[5] — reasons for this are unexplained in the medical literature but it could be that they are better able to modify ideas about themselves and the world — and that it often emerges months and even years after the traumatic event or situation.

In the last two years, numerous studies have been published that focus on PTG in Covid survivors. In one Italian study of seventy-one Covid ICU survivors who went on to have persistent symptoms of long Covid, 50 percent reported experiencing PTG six months after discharge, with 62 percent displaying "adaptive" coping strategies (defined as healthy approaches that center on problem-solving).[6] Growth was especially significant in the domain of renewed appreciation for life. In a large study conducted in Ghana of 381 patients hospitalized with Covid who experienced various mental health conditions after discharge, 53 percent described developing resilience after Covid, while 60 percent noted the presence of PTG.[7] Similar findings occurred in a Chinese investigation in which study subjects described wide-ranging benefits following their struggle with Covid and its aftermath, including reassessing key priorities in their life, better relationships with others, a new willingness to help others, and noticeable personal growth, defined as increased maturity and a more enriched life.

As the studies above demonstrate, the broadly observed phenomenon of PTG can occur in people living with long Covid, and many long haulers have experienced growth in their lives due to hard lessons learned while battling adversities and navigating their new existence. This, in turn, can offer hope and purpose. It's important to clarify that the possibility of post-traumatic growth does not negate the deep physical and emotional suffering that can accompany trauma or challenging situations in people's lives, nor does it mean that traumatic events are good. Instead, it is an acknowledgment that personal transformation may arise from the struggle and that great suffering may be a catalyst for growth.

FIVE AREAS OF GROWTH

Post-traumatic growth may manifest in various ways, but research suggests that people usually experience it in five different areas in their lives.

Deeper Appreciation for Life

One humid October evening, my wife, Michelle, and I, and two of our best friends, were sitting under the stars on the highest hilltop in Nashville, listening to music at Bluebird on the Mountain, an outdoor concert known, at the time, only to locals. It had been a week of difficult diagnoses at the clinic and several emotional sessions with patients, and I was just beginning to shift my focus to my evening out when the singers on stage belted out "Live Like You Were Dying." Though I'd heard this towering single by country singer Tim McGraw many times, it suddenly struck me that it was a paean to PTG if ever I'd heard one— the story of a man in the prime of life who receives a terminal cancer diagnosis and reevaluates his existence in the knowledge that his time here will be brief. In appreciating life, he no longer takes anything for granted, but pursues new passions and interests with gusto (skydiving, mountain climbing, bull riding) and makes changes to carve out a different way forward (through forgiveness and reading the "good book"). I sat in the half-darkness, mesmerized by the lyrics, wanting to find a way to incorporate some of what I was feeling into the care of my patients.

Some of my patients who have survived a severe case of acute Covid, who may have been in the ICU, and who continue to struggle with ongoing symptoms of long Covid have felt similarly grateful. They've started to look at life through a lens of deep appreciation. I'm thinking, as I write, of Laura, who was the manager of a retail drug store before she developed significant problems with neuropathy and cognitive impairment after a lengthy course of critical illness due to Covid. Life prior to her infection was fast paced with long hours spent at work, often putting out fires, juggling multiple tasks, and trying to stay a step or two ahead of the corporate office's expectations. Now she can't imagine how she used to handle it. She has quit her job and is working part time from home as a telemarketer, taking it slow. It's not what she envisioned nor is it what she wanted but she's come to appreciate the time she can spend with her young son and husband and with her hands in the earth in their small yard. She worries about the cut in the family income but with the babysitter expense gone and a fledgling vegetable garden in the works, she's determined to be thankful for what they have. "I keep my sights on my family," she says, "and on the hummingbirds that flit between the canna lilies in the garden."

Greater Openness to New Possibilities

For some, challenging life events can result in a desire or the necessity to change the way life was previously lived. This might include cultivating new interests to replace older ones that are no longer accessible or finding a new life path.

Samantha is in her late thirties, the mother of three young children, and previously a physicist who worked for the federal government in a series of increasingly responsible jobs. She developed Covid early in the first wave of the pandemic and, while many of her friends had similar experiences and seemed to get better, she never did. Now, she's been out of the workforce for a long while due to bone-crushing fatigue, which sometimes dissipates for a day or two but never really leaves, and a vast array of hard-to-explain symptoms that seem to be getting worse. She's doubtful that she will ever return to her previous job or her previous life. Dinners out with friends and family walks in the beautiful countryside near her house are impossible for her now, and she has spent a lot of time wishing she could turn back the clock. Her life is hard and littered with challenges that sometimes seem to threaten to engulf her, yet, in the midst of it all, she's managed to find a new way forward and sense of purpose—advocacy.

A former member of her college debate team, Samantha is thoughtful, quick, and articulate, and when speaking about long Covid she communicates with the sincerity and authority that come from experience. She's spoken to local, national, and even a couple of international reporters, and continues to look for opportunities to tell her story in ways that empower others and educate the public at large about the ongoing needs of long haulers. Her emerging role as an advocate hasn't necessarily made her daily difficulties any less profound—she misses her job and still relies on her mother, partner, and friends for a patchwork of childcare and household support, and the interviews can sap her energy for hours and sometimes days—but this burgeoning interest is motivating, powerful, and important. It makes her feel competent and seen. She's grateful for the growth she's witnessed in herself, even as she finds ways to deal with her reality.

Personal Strength: Knowing That You Can Handle Difficult Things

In the unfolding of a difficult life situation, or in the aftermath, some people take stock of what they have endured and realize they are stronger than they could have ever imagined, and this can lead to an increased sense of self-reliance and inner confidence. One of my patients, Maria, a young Australian international aid worker, ended up in the ICU and lost several toes due to profound circulatory problems. A vibrant young woman, she spent more than a month in the hospital and developed severe PTSD. After her discharge, she isolated herself and had daily panic attacks and serious symptoms that left her unable to function or return to work and, eventually, led her to receive therapy.

Recently my colleague Dr. Carla Sevin and I received an email with a video attachment from Maria, sent to the ICU Recovery

Center. When we opened it and saw the footage, we both laughed, though tears were close, too. There was Maria, back in Australia, on a surfboard, riding a wave, looking fierce, untamed, and determined. Her accompanying email was winsome and thoughtful, and she closed it with a statement (emphasis mine) that inspires and motivates me still, "I hope this email can serve as a solace when the days in the ICU seem never ending— *some of us survive and, even better, thrive.*"

Maria's growth didn't happen overnight. In the first year after her discharge, even as her PTSD symptoms lessened, she had bouts of depression and long periods of self-doubt in which she crawled under the bedcovers and stayed there, wracked by feelings of anxiety. But she continued to show up for therapy via telehealth and started to find meditation helpful. She also discovered that when she put the details of her story down on paper, she could step away and view it from a distance, and, in the process, learn to think about it differently. In time, she found that she was healing, developing a reservoir of strength that she didn't think she had, and finding the courage to return, little by little, to activities that she had once loved. One of these was surfing, a hobby she had dabbled in previously and that now seemed to call to her— part adventurous, part terrifying. Even though three toes on her dominant foot were gone, a daily reminder of what she had endured, she kept at it, determined to stand on her board and catch a wave. "I knew that after everything I'd been through I could do it," she said to me. And she did. Now she is hoping that one day she can start a therapeutic surfing retreat to help others grow after difficult life events.

Closer Relationships

As people reassess their lives in the face of upheavals and trauma, they may look at their relationships and the ways that they relate to others. Recently, I met with Chris, a patient of mine, and his wife, Claire, at the ICU Recovery Center. In their mid-fifties and living in northern Georgia, Chris is a nurse at a small country hospital, while Claire is a social worker. Chris had spent more than two months in the ICU with Covid and was so weak when he arrived at a rehabilitation hospital that he could barely walk or hold a pencil. His medical journey was a difficult one, each piece of positive news offset, it seemed, by a complication, and the one constant in the process was Claire. She sat steadfastly by his side in the hospital room, supporting him and advocating on his behalf, and, when hospital protocols dictated that she couldn't, she sat hunched in her car in the parking lot, as close as she could get. Sometimes she cried for hours, though she would never admit this to Chris. When Chris finally made it home, while he struggled with significant cognitive dysfunction, his brain foggy and his memory unsure, there was one thing that was clear in his mind: he would never have made it without Claire.

Their marriage has carried them through many seasons over the past thirty years, and a few times they had thrown their hands up in futility, wondering whether it was time to go their separate ways. Sometimes Claire stayed too long at work and Chris grew frustrated, feeling like her commitment to her patients lessened her time with him. At times it felt like a minor miracle that they remained together and yet, as they sat together during their appointment, Chris held Claire's hand and talked through tears about his renewed love and profound gratitude for her and the terror he felt when he remembered how close they had come to divorcing just a few short years ago. "I didn't know how lucky I was," he said, shaking his head. The difference in their relationship, driven by Chris's realization of how lovingly Claire had cared for him—indeed, how much she *loved* him—and his newly discovered respect for her, was palpable. Claire said that she felt seen now and valued. That she didn't need to prove her love for Chris; it was a given. I watched them talking together, making plans for the week ahead, for Chris's appointments with his speech and language pathologist, a dinner for Claire with an old college friend, maybe a movie. They seemed in sync with each other.

A Spiritual Change

This might include a deepening of, or a shift in, a current belief system, or involvement with a new religion or belief system. Pulitzer Prize–winning war reporter Ernie Pyle is sometimes credited with saying, "there are no atheists in foxholes" (although some attribute the phrase to others) and while this quote is not strictly true as approximately[8] 2 percent of soldiers in the United States Armed Forces identify as atheists, it highlights the point that many people turn to religious faith or perhaps spirituality, more broadly, during times of great stress.

Over decades of working with survivors of critical illness and, more recently, with people with long Covid, I have often observed this change take place in people's lives. It unfolds in a variety of ways. Sometimes people experience an awakening of a long dormant faith or the faith they practice seems more urgent and personal. Some people may turn toward a new belief system that feels more in keeping with who they are now, and others may experience a transcendent spiritualty, a sense of oneness with the universe that leads to increased peace. Serious illness and devastating life events can shake people to the core, often leaving them feeling vulnerable, and some look to religion as a guide and a support.

One of my patients embraced Buddhism, feeling especially drawn to its philosophies of compassion, responsibility, and values in an impermanent world. Post-Covid fatigue and cognitive dysfunction had taken away his ability to drive and with it his volunteer work at an animal shelter, and now he is hoping to rebuild his life from what he describes as a solid foundation of faith. Another patient, Richard, a middle-aged accountant from Indiana, has struggled with multiple seizure-like episodes since contracting Covid and is now unable to work. He's distressed by his poor health, of course, and concerned about disability benefits, but he has also experienced a profound sense of serenity that is hard to explain. He is convinced that no matter how difficult things get, he's going to be okay because his life is part of an unfolding story that God is writing and shepherding. For him, his faith allows him to trust the process and to accept his life the way it is. For each person, the role of religion, spirituality, or belief in a higher power after trauma is unique.

DEVELOPING POST-TRAUMATIC GROWTH

I like to see my patients thrive, and I would very much like them to experience post-traumatic growth as I believe it can help considerably in managing an illness or condition. Usually, however, PTG arises organically and cannot be brought about by wishing it or trying to engineer its development. That said, I do regularly explore with patients, both in individual therapy sessions and in group treatment, the possibility that they could be experiencing post-traumatic growth. After considering whether raising the subject is appropriate, I aim to initiate questions thoughtfully, trying to meet my patients where they are and without an agenda. I'm acutely aware that positivity-tinged discussions can be perceived as tone deaf, or insensitive, as minimizing someone's struggles. In many cases, I don't say anything at all, and at other times, I tread carefully, engaging in a discussion only after a patient has raised the subject.

However, I always want to be open to the possibility of post-traumatic growth in my patients' lives and am guided in my approach by two beliefs. First, I think it unwise to assume that people who experience difficult situations are impacted exclusively in negative ways, and second, I've observed and continue to witness the ways that PTG has been at work in my life as I've learned to acknowledge, accept, and adapt to my OCD diagnosis. Over the years, I have experienced growth in two primary areas of my life: my relationships with others and spiritual change. I've always been quite a gregarious extrovert and enjoy relationships with people, and, more recently, I've found that my friendships have grown in intimacy. I'm more willing to share my inner self, especially with close friends. When texting my childhood friend and high school football teammate, Bob, I regularly end our conversation with the words "I love you" (I love you, Bob!!!) and on dates with my wife, Michelle, I'm less inclined to talk about the weather and more interested in talking about things of consequence that lead to deepened bonds, even if the conversations are not always easy. With my faith, always a central feature of my life, I have become less attached to the rational, no longer needing tidy explanations, and feeling comfortable and often in awe of mysteries and paradoxes that I can't—and don't need to—clarify.

While it may not be possible to choose whether you experience post-traumatic growth, there are certain conditions, based on my clinical experience, that may help you to foster and develop it:

Cultivate an Attitude of Openness

Try to see your struggle with long Covid in a different way, remaining open to the idea that this journey, as difficult as it is, can foster new insights and contribute to your growth over time. When my psychologist first raised the possibility that my battle with OCD might give rise to good things, to positive developments in my life, I took great affront at the idea and closed myself off to everything she said. Eventually, as I let the idea percolate, I became very *slightly* open to the possibility, though I still dismissed it, but by cracking the door just a little and being willing to consider her words I was able to let big changes start to work.

Try to crack the door and think about adopting a stance of curiosity about your experiences that may not be intuitive, may not make sense, and could even be distressing.

Ask yourself questions about the meaning of your trauma and its impact on you. This "deliberate rumination," as Tedeschi and Calhoun refer to it, starts with a willingness to entertain the idea that such an exercise could be valuable and, as you begin to make sense of events, can lead to PTG.

Share Your Story with Other People

One of the obvious consequences of Covid-19 has been social isolation and disengagement from others and from shared social spaces where relationships often happen. Many days I look out of the narrow window in my office onto the breakroom in our office suite, and I'm reminded that no one is eating there together anymore because many people are working at home. I miss the casual conversations that took place while waiting in line to use the microwave or standing around the proverbial watercooler that often seemed to prompt deeper connections and disclosures. While some are not having these interactions because they are working remotely, millions of people with long Covid around the world are no longer in the workforce at all. Even in neighborhoods, community centers, places of worship, and schools, isolation abounds, and we often have to work harder than we once did to connect with others. It can be especially crucial for those going through difficult life experiences.

Multiple research studies on PTG show that it can develop in the context of close relationships,[9] especially with those undergoing similar experiences, people who can empathize, encourage, and share their stories and strategies, including how to reappraise their situation.[10,11] Many of my patients have found support groups — in person, on Zoom, or online — very helpful, and I offer more details in Chapter 8. Likewise, I have seen firsthand the way that long haulers provide one another encouragement, guidance, and solidarity in the peer support groups that my colleagues and I lead each week. They appear to provide an atmosphere conducive to the development of post-traumatic growth.

Try to find environments and situations in which you can get together with like-minded people and safely explore the narratives you've developed around your particular story.

As you share your story and listen to others' experiences, consider whether there may be other perspectives or alternative ways to manage your struggles.

Be aware that sharing your story may be a difficult emotional experience *and* that this raw honesty can lead you to developing deeper bonds with others.

Lean In to Healthy Coping Strategies

Several useful insights stand out in the scientific literature on how coping strategies can affect the development of PTG. In general, tools that promote post-traumatic growth help people view difficulties and setbacks more positively, encourage adaptability, and assign meaning to challenges. These strategies may be helpful for you:

Acceptance Coping

At its essence, acceptance coping means accepting (rather than avoiding or denying) that a challenging life situation is real and must be addressed. My clinical observations fit with this finding. The long haulers I work with who are able to look directly at the difficulties in their lives, who don't deny them or sugarcoat them but see the full magnitude of their challenges and can find the grit to talk about and engage them, often experience post-traumatic growth.

Carl, a middle school librarian in his mid-forties, developed severe panic attacks and experienced dissociative episodes after recovering from Covid and ended up being hospitalized for a brief time to help stabilize his mental health. Shaken by the sudden turn of events in his life, Carl was terrified by what it might mean for his future, and while part of him didn't really want to find out, he knew that he needed to pursue treatment, probably therapy, which was far beyond his comfort zone. As I meet with him weekly, I continue to be struck by his willingness to acknowledge the challenges that his symptoms pose, to face the possibility that he may have to navigate a mental health diagnosis for the rest of his life, and to summon the courage necessary to cope. He drives from Kentucky to the ICU Recovery Center to see me for weekly individual psychotherapy sessions and engages in extensive and exhausting visits to psychiatrists, following trial-and-error efforts with multiple psychotropic medications to find one that works and often having to keep panic attacks at bay. His ability to "lean in" and address his debilitating symptoms is beginning to help him understand and manage them, and to find a way to live with them. In time, his hard work may lead to personal growth. I hope so.

- Try to face the full scope of your difficulties, no matter how hard it may seem.
- Though it may be terrifying, aim to stay the course of treatment.
- Surround yourself with supportive people to help buoy your spirits.

Avoidance Coping

The vast amount of psychological literature on coping is consistent in demonstrating that avoidance is an ineffective strategy, for the most part, and often makes problems worse. As such, it is a coping mechanism that I would rarely encourage my patients to adopt. Yet there are situations in which avoidance coping can be helpful in the short term.

Shown in multiple studies to be associated with the development of PTG, avoidance coping refers to stepping away from traumatic and triggering thoughts and activities when they become too upsetting. It may seem that this method would conflict with exposure therapies that help patients face their traumatic experiences, but the key here is timing, balance, and dosage. Avoidance coping, often effective in the temporary reduction of distress, can be a healthy approach when paired with a commitment to face stressors when the time is right. Colette, one of the patients in my long Covid support group, recently started reading *The Body Keeps the Score,* a classic and groundbreaking work by psychiatrist Bessel van der Kolk, on the way that trauma is stored in the body. As Colette delved into the book, she found herself feeling overwhelmed and frantic, unable to focus, or to get herself to her job. It seemed as if the book were written about her. She made the decision to put the book away for a time, and yet she didn't want to ignore what it was telling her—it felt important. She decided to commit to return to the book when she had found a therapist who could help her with her unresolved trauma and support her as she coped with the many thoughts and feelings that she believed reading would provoke. In doing so, Colette applied the strategy of avoidance coping and combined it with acceptance coping.

In contrast, one of my long Covid patients, Clarence, a truck driver and former army infantryman, so desperately wanted to be free from the daily assaults on his well-being caused by PTSD that he moved too quickly and undermined his own progress. He had developed PTSD after a prolonged stay in the ICU, and while his indomitable will had helped him succeed in the military, his determination to combat his PTSD was less helpful. He forced himself to talk about painful memories of his hospital experience and to engage in "exposures" such as returning to the emergency department where he had been admitted, wanting to face his illness head-on. Unfortunately, he developed more distress than growth and healing, and set himself back in his recovery. Like many people, Clarence had associated going slow with his treatment or pacing himself as signs of weakness, and while it can be hard to wait to begin to feel better, a combination of avoidance coping and acceptance coping can be the most effective strategy.

Be willing to pace yourself in your treatment. Sometimes it is a quicker way to see results.

Acknowledge that dealing with life-changing events is difficult and that sometimes a break can be beneficial. It doesn't mean that you've stopped moving forward in your recovery—it is part of the process.

Positive Reappraisal

This strategy refers to the ability to view or consider negative events in a more positive way by using techniques such as reframing or reinterpreting. One of my patients, Amy, has been using this method recently and it is helping her feel more encouraged about her current situation. A life-threatening case of Covid-19 and multiple ongoing symptoms caused her to retire early from her job as a logistics director at a large auto parts manufacturer, and in the months that followed, she spent a lot of time looking back on her work, feeling forlorn and angry as she thought about how much she had enjoyed having a job and all it had represented for her. Now she felt lost without it, her days endless and meaningless. She worried about the drastic decrease in income and fought back feelings of being a failure. On the phone with her sister one evening, Amy lamented again the loss of her job and heard her sister respond, "I'm so sorry. I just hadn't realized that you loved it so much." For a moment, Amy paused. Had she loved it?

Later that night, Amy began to remember her job in a different way, not as an abstract entity that gave her life meaning, but as the job it really was, one that had frustrated her much of the time and had infringed on her life in countless ways. She recalled the relentless demands, expectations that could not possibly be met, long hours that had become increasingly taxing as she grew older, the accompanying stress, family celebrations missed, vacations postponed, the high blood pressure that worried her family members as well as her physician who, on a few occasions, had told her gently if bluntly, "If you keep working like this, it's going to kill you." As Amy continued to reflect, talking her thoughts over in therapy, she realized that while losing her job was painful, it may have also been a gift—one that saved her life. With this positive reappraisal, she was able to start thinking about what her job loss meant to her, and how she might find other ways to fill the void it had left in her life, to find meaning elsewhere, and to begin to find a new way forward, compatible with her body's new limitations.

Be open to the idea that there may be a different story about yourself or your life that can give you an alternative perspective and new ideas for moving forward.

Try journaling to reframe narratives, looking at your pre-Covid life through a new lens. Is it really the way you remember it? What about your new reality? Does the way you present it reflect the whole truth?

As a teenager, I wanted to be a great athlete. It was my primary goal when I woke up in the morning; on summer afternoons, when I charged up and down a dusty football practice field dragging an old tire behind me, and when I turned into bed and listened to my beloved Detroit Tigers baseball games on my portable radio. I had motivational sayings and posters plastered all over my room, taped onto the walls and ceiling and, in my wallet, I carried the granddaddy of them all—a square of paper that I turned to again and again that simply said "Whatever doesn't kill you makes you stronger." I probably had no idea who Friedrich Nietzsche was in those days, but I uttered this quote many times over as I prepared for hard wrestling practices and workouts that promised to be exhausting.

I've evolved over the past forty years, and now the aphorism strikes me as abrupt, overly certain, and uncaring as I think about thousands of patients who have been utterly broken, not emboldened, by dealing with unthinkably hard events in their lives. In my clinical practice, I try to tend to my patients with kindness, gentleness, respect, and compassion without the glorification of suffering. And yet, I do believe, and you may agree, that in some circumstances, beauty does arise from ashes, and, though we may wish that the ashes had never appeared, it can be helpful to make room for, or even to seek out, the beauty. By being curious, open, and reflective, sharing stories of suffering with others, and embracing ways of coping that promote our growth, it can be possible to, at least, encourage transformation, even amid long Covid struggles.

As I draw the chapter to a close, here are some questions to help you think about the place of post-traumatic growth in your life and how to recognize its presence or foster its development:

- Do you have a greater appreciation for life?
- Have you changed your priorities about what is important in life?

- Do you have new interests?
- Are you committed to changing things that need changing?
- Have you been surprised by your strength?
- Do you have a greater understanding of your resilience?
- Do you feel closer to others?
- Are you more willing to be vulnerable and express your emotions?
- Have your beliefs changed?
- Do you have a new or greater sense of spirituality?

CHAPTER 8

CONNECTING WITH OTHERS:
Harnessing the Power of Social Engagement

Since the beginning of the pandemic, I've cared for and communicated with countless people living with long Covid, and, as many others have observed, they don't fit a tidy narrative. Their symptoms can differ hugely, manifesting to varying degrees for unpredictable lengths of time, and impacting their lives in unique ways. Long haulers come from all walks of life—low, middle, and high socioeconomic circumstances, diverse races and ethnicities, and across a wide range of educational backgrounds. They cut across gender and age groups and reside in cities, suburbs, and rural enclaves around the world. Before they became ill, some ran marathons or swam laps daily at the YMCA, while others toyed with eating better and walking more, and still others had premorbid and chronic conditions of various kinds. In short, they are different in the ways that all of us, as humans, are different.

However, in my exchanges with long haulers, whether patients or people in our support groups, or others who reach me via email or social media, I have found, as conversations turn vulnerable, one constant that slices through everything else. Many people living with long Covid feel physically isolated and/or emotionally lonely, even those living with others. For some, it is a surprise when they say the words out loud and for others, it is a relief. We are a social species, and though we may try to deny it, we need other people in our lives, especially when we are mired in difficult circumstances.

In this chapter, I explore the roles of isolation and social engagement in living with long Covid, including their effects on health, and provide support and guidance in bringing shared activities into your life.

FACTORS LEADING TO ISOLATION AND LONELINESS

Isolation is a physical separation from other people, and social isolation refers to an absence of relationships with others. Both can lead to the experience of loneliness, a deep ache of sadness, emptiness, and rejection. People can feel lonely even in the presence of others. There are many reasons for isolation among long haulers, some intentional—often for reasons of health and safety—some imposed by limitations caused by long Covid symptoms, and others that may have made sense at one time and have now become habits.

With Covid variants still circulating and most mandatory restrictions such as masking and social distancing a thing of the past, for many people with long Covid a certain degree of physical disengagement from society is important and prioritized as a way of helping to ensure their health and well-being. This might mean not having people over to visit, or not seeing friends or family, especially at larger gatherings. Many long haulers have opted for working from home, or for online classes, or telehealth visits, whenever possible, to keep themselves safe and to decrease the likelihood of reinfection with Covid. For those who might like, or need, to leave the house, physical disability, often in the form of intense fatigue, shortness of breath, or vertigo, can make it difficult to do so. Driving may no longer be an option, taking public transportation could be unrealistic, and depending on the kindness of others may not be a long-term solution.

Cognitive deficits can also be a limitation in engaging with others, contributing to decisions made by many long haulers to stay home rather than participate in social events. Some grow self-conscious about their reduced ability to effectively respond to others, to think on their feet, and to track conversations. One of my patients has significant processing-speed delays. When people ask him questions, he feels as if he is operating in slow motion, taking what seems like minutes to answer and, in the process, experiencing intense embarrassment. Socializing is now uncomfortable for him. Another patient worries about forgetting the names of people she has known for years, or not recognizing them at all.

In many cases, psychological concerns play a role in increasing isolation among those living with long Covid. Quite a few of my patients avoid hospitals, clinics, and other healthcare settings, as they find these environments triggering. Some patients who experience panic attacks worry about having one in public and so try to avoid leaving home, especially alone, as much as possible. Others find that their anxiety has been exacerbated by Covid, and the thought of going to class, attending an event, or mingling with large crowds leaves them paralyzed with fear.

Many of my patients have told me that even when surrounded by others, they may feel disconnected, misunderstood, or discounted by people who have moved on from the pandemic and think they should, too. Or they may be wrapped up in feelings of shame, acutely aware of the often stark differences between who they are now and who they were before. One of my patients recounted a friend's words—"You're no fun anymore!"—and talked about her social circle growing smaller and smaller. "You find out who your real friends are," she added ruefully.

There are myriad reasons for isolation and loneliness. You may recognize yourself in some of the scenarios I've mentioned, or you may have experienced others. All are easily understood and easy to empathize with — sometimes my OCD has made me stay home, too. Unfortunately, decades of research and vast clinical experience show that isolation is unhelpful at best and often profoundly harmful. In contrast, a different way of living and interacting with the world, one marked by some form of social contact, has far-reaching benefits for our health.

RESEARCH

Recent scientific research suggests that our brain considers social engagement a basic biological need, in the same way that our bodies require water, food, and air to survive.[1] It makes sense then that when this need is not fulfilled, there can be detrimental effects to our health. Multiple studies show that social isolation is a key contributor to the development of many mental health conditions and concerns, including anxiety,[2] depression,[3] substance use disorder,[4] and suicidal ideation,[5] but it is not only mental health that suffers. Research has also linked it to negative impacts on physical health, leading to high blood pressure,[6,7] obesity,[8,9] greater risk of heart disease and stroke,[10] sleep problems,[11] and, in one large examination of nearly 600,000 adults, a heightened risk of premature death (increasing in white people by up to 84 percent and doubling in Black people).[12] Indeed, in a recent meta-analysis that gathered and analyzed the results of existing studies, researchers found that social isolation is as harmful to our health as smoking fifteen cigarettes a day and twice as damaging to physical health as morbid obesity.[13]

Cognitive functioning, already vulnerable in many people with long Covid, also erodes, with evidence suggesting that social isolation contributes to neuropsychological difficulties. In one of the definitive studies on the topic, a 2022 investigation that followed 400,000 middle-aged British people for up to twelve years, social isolation was associated with a 26 percent increased risk of dementia as well as decreased brain volume, an undesirable outcome usually due to the death of neurons, often indicative of accelerated brain aging and a sign of cognitive problems to come.[14]

Social engagement, on the other hand, confers far-reaching benefits. Studies show that it protects against the development and worsening of many chronic conditions such as diabetes[15] and heart disease[16] and is associated with increased longevity.[17] It can improve mental health and helps prevent mental health problems—so much so that people engaged in making regular connections with others are up to 50 percent happier,[18] experience significantly less depression,[19] and, as described in a six-country study of 33,000 people, self-reported a better quality of life.

Social interaction fosters a deep sense of belonging,[20] which, in turn, has been shown to result in positive outcomes, including improved confidence, stronger relationships, and a greater sense of collaboration with others.[21] Importantly, social engagement slows the rate of cognitive decline and, in some cases, leads to improved cognitive functioning and increased cognitive reserve (think of this as a cognitive muscle that creates a buffer against the development of dementia). In an investigation published in 2021, in which nearly three hundred participants from the Health, Aging and Body Composition Study received a sophisticated brain scan using diffusion tensor imaging, data showed that those who had greater social interaction and increased participation in activities had healthier gray matter than those who were less socially engaged, especially in key brain regions implicated in dementia.[22]

THE INSIDIOUS CREEP OF ISOLATION

As I've noted, there are often considerable obstacles that prevent long haulers from engaging with the outside world. In many cases, there may be so many other elements to juggle in navigating a new illness that it may not be possible to prioritize social engagement at all. My patient, Sierra, is a good example.

In her words, Sierra, a young entrepreneur originally from Casper, Wyoming, was once "the life of the party." Lively, dynamic, outgoing, and a natural connector of people, she enjoyed spending summer weekends at the lake with her friends, days that often turned into long evenings of food and fun. Her story of surviving Covid is one of dominos falling. After a severe acute case that kept her at home and in bed for several weeks, she thought she was through the worst until intense fatigue and gastrointestinal issues developed. Standing up brought on waves of vertigo and vomiting, confining her to a lying-down position. Work was impossible, and with no access to disability insurance (her employer had not offered it) and family members unsupportive, financial problems soon set in. She tried valiantly to resolve them, searching for some kind of work to do from home, living on ramen for weeks, even selling possessions until there was nothing left to sell.

Even as some of her symptoms started to abate, she found excuses to avoid going out, worried that her friends would choose a restaurant she couldn't afford, inviting them over instead for the cheapest pizza she could find. Eventually, as her savings ran out, she moved to a tiny apartment on the edge of town, on the corner, as she said in her inimitable way, of Hell and Hell. It was that or move back in with her parents. She stays home alone most days watching TV, too ashamed to reach out to friends and too upset with family members who lost patience with her long ago, telling her it was time to "suck it up, buttercup." When measured on a calendar, she is not so far removed from August afternoons on a pontoon boat and nights spent around the fire pit with her friends but now, when she thinks about those days, they seem like they were a lifetime ago. Her slide into isolation and loneliness is surprising to her, but one that she doesn't know how to fix. She sees it as just one more insurmountable problem.

SUPPORT GROUPS

For many long haulers like Sierra, a support group (in person, virtual, or online) can be a good first step toward becoming social. Participation in a healing community of people, a safe space in which to share stories and challenges can foster a sense of belonging while decreasing shame, stigma, and isolation. I have seen this firsthand in my work over the years with survivors of critical illness and, more recently, in our long Covid support groups.

Almost a decade ago, as I had in-depth conversations with ICU survivors, both at our clinic and in their homes, I learned about their day-to-day lives and how they were affected by the aftermath of critical illness. Perhaps the most enduring insight was that my patients felt deeply alone. I began to be aware of the army of advocates both in middle Tennessee, where I live, and around the world who host 5K fun runs to raise breast cancer awareness, bring attention to the needs of people with multiple sclerosis, and hold support groups for caregivers of Alzheimer's disease, among others, and I was struck by the fact that ICU survivors had no one to champion their cause—and no one to turn to and share their experience with. Not quite sure what we were doing but hoping to be helpful, we decided to start our own ICU survivor support group at the CIBS Center.

We put out the word that we would be meeting weekly on the second floor of a local church and waited. For a while, my co-leader and I were the only ones who showed up but, in time, people came, and soon we had eight or ten regular members, telling their stories, finding kinship, and building connections that were deeply transforming. We hadn't known what to expect and were happy to let the sessions develop organically, soon seeing that the group was better called a community, a place where people of diverse ages, life experiences, and backgrounds came together for emotional support and to build relationships that I soon realized would become lifelong bonds.

We were early adopters of a virtual format, recognizing that using communication platforms such as Zoom would allow people from farther afield to participate, and would be more inclusive of people with disabilities. One day, a new support group member, Kipp, who lived three hundred miles away from Nashville in a mountain "holler," shared that he had been diagnosed with an aneurysm but needed a second opinion before embarking on a potentially risky procedure. Seeing a neurosurgeon at Vanderbilt was an option, but he didn't drive and paying for transportation was prohibitively expensive. Even now, I'm struggling to describe the pride and amazement I felt when two group members told him they would drive to his tiny village, pick him up, take him to his appointment, cover all his expenses, and return him home afterward. I know that the practical help was much needed and appreciated by Kipp, but the emotional support, true connection, and acknowledgment was lifesaving. The support group became one of the most well-used tools in our care of patients after their ICU stay.

In mid-2020, my longtime colleague Amy Kiehl and I decided to start a similar support group for people with long Covid. We realized that long haulers had few therapeutic resources available to them. In a very short time, people started attending our group, first from middle Tennessee, then from neighboring states and across the United States, Canada, and, later, even from Europe. (Patients from Nashville are now in the minority.) In just a few months, our first group was bursting at the seams, routinely filled with well over twenty people, too many for the group to be optimally therapeutic. We created a second group and a third and began to refer Covid ICU survivors to our long-standing ICU support group.

Currently, our support groups serve approximately sixty patients a week, with a waiting list of between thirty and fifty patients at any particular time, a fact that speaks to the unmet need for community and support among Covid survivors and their families. As we work to increase our capacity to create additional groups, Amy and I refer people to other support groups, and, as demand continues to rise, we consult with other healthcare systems in the US and around the world, advising them on developing similar models of care.

Initially, we planned our groups to be instructive, led by two mental health professionals who would teach participants a wide range of coping strategies such as concepts from Acceptance and Commitment

Therapy and cognitive rehabilitation tools such as Goal Management Training. While attendees benefited from learning specific techniques—e.g., how to break complicated problems into manageable parts and how to practice mindfulness—they consistently told us that acquiring skills, no matter how helpful, was not their primary need. Rather, as *Teen Vogue* writer Fortesa Latifi wrote after visiting us and sitting in on a support group session, "Perhaps the biggest benefit of the support groups is just being in the company of other people who are going through the same thing as you are."

I have seen, and patients have confirmed, that the value of a support group is its function as a safe place, as somewhere to be understood, seen, and validated, as a family of sorts for people going through something difficult. The support group is a good way to become social and, as many groups have no prohibition against communication outside of the group, members often stay in touch during the week, integrating their lives in tender and nurturing ways.

For many months now, I have seen Sierra participate in countless sessions with one of our support groups, showing up on her Zoom screen each week, and I've felt intense pride in her as she has moved from social isolation to active social engagement. It didn't happen overnight—it rarely does. At first, she was reluctant to join the group, but she said she would give it a try. Since then, week after week, she has sat in front of her camera, leaning in and telling her story, embracing it with courage as she finds her voice. She still lives in her apartment on the corner of Hell and Hell but as she listens to and engages with others, she's started to modify her thinking and, by extension, the way she feels about her situation. No one is judging or shaming her here and so she feels less inclined to do so herself. She sees that many people in the group are living in environments every bit as difficult as hers, making her plight not less challenging but, perhaps, more possible to accept.

In following the guidance of fellow group members who have found ways to extend their footprint as they've pushed back against isolation, she adopted a senior dog and together they go for slow walks, a few steps farther each time. She enjoys getting outside a couple of times a day and the impromptu conversations with other dog owners along the way. Over the weeks, she has watched with curiosity as many of her peers have treated themselves with kindness and acceptance, and she has started doing the same, no longer speaking to herself in critical and acerbic tones over progress that has moved too slowly.

Since the "wheels came off the car," as Sierra likes to say in her distinctive Western drawl, she has spent much of her time ruminating— about her lost job, the friends who have let her down, and her estranged family. But this dynamic is starting to change. With the help and care of support group members, she has been reminded that she has much to offer.

JOINING A SUPPORT GROUP

If you are interested in joining a long Covid support group, whether in person, virtually, or online, there are a variety of options for doing so. Many groups are available to access via an internet connection, which removes the barrier of finding a way to get there in person.

In-Person/Virtual Support Groups

These groups are often affiliated with hospital networks or post-Covid care clinics (PCCC) and may require a formal referral from a health-care provider. In many instances, however, you can call the intake coordinator and self-refer. If you are working with a PCP knowledge-able about long Covid, or already have an appointment with a doctor, or a healthcare team at a PCCC, they may be able to point you to resources or help you to find a group. Otherwise, you may have to phone different PCCCs to inquire about availability. Survivor Corps, self-described as the "largest grassroots movement in America dedicated to actively ending this pandemic," maintains a helpful, regularly updated (though not all-encompassing) list and dynamic map of long Covid clinics on its website (survivorcorps.com/pccc).

Many of these support groups follow a similar format to those we offer at Vanderbilt, including one led by my psychology colleague Dr. Erin Hall at Geisinger Medical Center in Pennsylvania, or the in-person group at Bon Secours medical center in upstate South Carolina. Facilitated by mental health professionals, they typically have fewer than twenty people at a time. In some cases, they focus on the acquisition of coping skills and education about conditions such as cognitive impairment and PTSD, and in other instances, group members direct the conversation. These groups may, at first glance, have fewer opportunities for interaction with others as numbers are more limited, but it can be easier for deeper relationships to flourish over time as group members get to know one another and care for one another's well-being. In addition, there are usually opportunities to benefit from the guidance of professionals who often become partners in care and are available to answer questions and concerns in between sessions. In general, most support groups are provided as a free service for anyone who wants to join, though each group will likely have its own policies. Some may have waitlists.

If finding a support group for long Covid survivors is difficult, other options are to find a group that supports those living with chronic illness or, if appropriate, to participate in a mental health support group, both designed to bring people with diverse stories and challenges together to provide camaraderie, connection, and even accountability.

Online Groups

There are many different support groups available online for long haulers and a simple way to find them is through an online search. It may lead you to one of the many groups on Facebook, such as the Long Covid Support Group, a private group that is open to all and currently has more than 55,000 members from around the world, or to the Body Politic Support Group another well-run, practical, and valuable resource for patients impacted by long Covid.

In general, online support groups aim to provide a sense of family and community, connect members with others who are going through a similar experience, offer resources, and allow members to discuss symptoms and treatments (many groups have rules that forbid sharing of unsubstantiated health advice). In addition, some also encourage—or provide opportunities for—members to mobilize and advocate for more treatments and medical research and be involved in clinical trials.

For example, Body Politic, originally founded as a queer feminist wellness collective in 2018, launched their Covid-19 support group for patients and family members in the early days of the pandemic and sees raising awareness about chronic illness, disability, and inequity in healthcare as a core part of its mission. The group offers discussions on many aspects of living with long Covid and chronic illness to many thousands around the globe with the possibility for smaller group interactions, specialized group membership (such as LGBTQ+ or parents of Covid survivors), and patient advocacy work through offshoot organizations.

Some support groups target more specialized populations such as the Black, Indigenous, and People of Color (BIPOC) Women's Long Hauler Support Group, a community of about four hundred people who meet virtually, bonded by shared experiences, especially of being marginalized and minimized by healthcare providers who fail to meet or appreciate their needs. You'll likely find an online group that works for you.

Larger online groups give patients (and sometimes family members) the opportunity to dip their toes into social engagement anonymously and on their own terms before deciding whether they would like to be more involved, perhaps in local groups that may even meet in person.

While some long Covid clinics require a positive Covid test to access treatment (though this is changing), such requirements do not exist for support groups. As you consider the relative benefits and drawbacks of different kinds of support groups and weigh these against your needs, be aware that you don't have to make either/or decisions. Many patients in small professionally led groups are involved in larger online communities, too, and find both helpful and meaningful in different and complementary ways.

HOW TO GET THE MOST OUT OF A SUPPORT GROUP

As we've seen, support groups can be a valuable resource, and many people who consider joining them want to ensure that they are as beneficial as possible. Reaping the rewards of a support group can be achieved in several ways. I'll outline four options here:

Active Engagement

Recently, I met one of my patients for an individual therapy session. In his late forties, Rudy retired from his job as a salesman and suffers the persistent effects of cognitive impairment that developed after a mild case of Covid last year. He is a member of one of our long Covid support groups and, over the last few months, I have watched him transition from a relatively passive group participant to an active one, turning into one of his group's leaders.

In our sessions each week, after providing any relevant news or updates, we invite group members to share whatever might be in their hearts. Often there is a silence that can last thirty seconds or more and if no one volunteers, Rudy jumps in with the same intensity and enthusiasm that he told me he used to have when he was a basketball center on his high school team in a small town just north of Nashville.

During our session, he told me he worried that he was monopolizing the group (he isn't) and he wanted to make sure other people had time to share (they do) but he noted that he was on a mission to derive as much benefit as he possibly could from every group meeting and to try to make the group as helpful to others as it could possibly be. Recalling his glory days on the basketball court, fighting with other players in the paint three decades earlier, he told me that if there was a lane, he was going to take it. I've watched him do this gracefully and repeatedly — to his benefit and that of the group.

Active engagement:

- Listen to others in the group and try to affirm their experiences.
- If you have something to share, please do so.
- Ask questions to clarify.
- Invite others to respond. Perhaps you could say, "Has that happened to anyone else?"
- Be encouraging — nodding your head is a way of showing support.

Vulnerability

If Rudy is an example of active participation, Camille represents vulnerability, a way of relating defined well by influential writer and researcher Brené Brown as "uncertainty, risk, and emotional exposure." A recent Covid survivor, Camille has been unable to stay active since contracting the virus, as constant exhaustion keeps her housebound and, as a consequence of her more sedentary lifestyle, she has gained a significant amount of weight.

In a recent group session, she shared that while at a visit with her PCP, she learned that she now has Type II diabetes, a lifelong fear of hers as she had seen both her parents struggle with it. She cried as she recounted her sadness over this painful development, one more insult in a long line of losses and disappointments. Afterward, she apologized, worried that her disclosure might overwhelm and even repel people or add a negative vibe to the session, bringing others down. To her great surprise, quite the opposite happened. People responded in turn, thanking her for sharing, volunteering to talk about their struggles, and revealing glimpses of their private pain. Everyone in the group drew closer as a result.

Vulnerability:

- Sharing your story can foster deeper connections—so be prepared to tell your story.
- Open up as it feels comfortable for you—and don't feel pressured.
- Be accepting and kind to others sharing details that may take courage. You could say, "That must have been hard to tell us."
- Think about when the timing might be right. It is usually best to know the group a little before you share something very personal.
- Know that telling personal stories can bring difficult emotions—and that is okay.

Preparation

Active engagement and vulnerability can go a long way toward turning your experience in a support group into a rich one, and a little preparation beforehand can make a huge difference. Unfortunately, many long haulers experience problems with executive functioning, and struggles with technology, attention to detail, and memory deficits are common and can lead to a frustrating and unsatisfactory experience with a support group. Often our patients have difficulties using online communication platforms, especially with turning on—or off—video and audio features, typing in chat boxes, as well as carefully reading email instructions and finding and using links to join online sessions. Time management and organization can create problems as well. Sometimes, our members lose track of time and miss sessions or log in at the wrong time or forget to charge computers and disappear in the middle of calls.

Preparation:

- Recognize that something, in this case a support group meeting, is important, and prioritize it.

- Make a note of the meeting on calendars and set alerts.
- Think about what is needed to show up on time for the meeting and ask for help in doing so. Do you need a reminder or a bit of persuasion? It could come from family members, friends, other group members, or from the group's organizers.
- Write a list or have sticky notes that remind you how to prepare for the meeting, including charging your computer, etc.
- Try out your technology before the meeting. Ask for help if needed. Group organizers are often happy to troubleshoot problems and to have practice runs before a meeting to help members feel confident in their ability to attend.

Showing Up

While familiarity with technology is important and planning and timeliness often contribute to the best possible experience, it is equally important to avoid all-or-nothing thinking. If you can attend just part of a support group because you couldn't get your video to work for the first half, it is better than not attending at all.

I was reminded of this lesson just this week. Michelle and I recently dropped our son off at college and, around the same time, our other son moved away from Nashville. As often happens during major life changes, my symptoms of OCD accelerated a little and so I scheduled an appointment with my psychologist for a check-in. I underestimated how long it would take me to get to her office, and by the time I arrived, I was thirty minutes late for my hour-long session. However, the thirty remaining minutes of therapy were the best thirty minutes of my week.

Showing up:

- Meet with your group however and whenever you can, as it is the only way they can be supportive of you (and you of them).
- Trust that your fellow support group members want you to be there.
- Know that the group leaders want you to be there.

- Even if you arrive late, the session can still be valuable.
- It's okay to show up with your camera off if that sometimes feels better for you.
- No one will mind if the backdrop behind you is messy, or if you are at a standing desk or lying under a blanket on a couch.
- You'll feel glad that you showed up.

MAKING SOCIAL CONNECTIONS

While joining a support group works well for many long haulers, it is not for everyone, nor is it the only kind of social engagement that people may yearn for. In speaking with Covid survivors and with people who feel isolated and derailed by the effects of the pandemic more generally, I sense that we are craving connection but aren't quite sure how to go about it. Many of us are still wary about social contact with others, and the idea of gathering as we used to may no longer be appealing or possible. In addition to limitations imposed by medical symptoms, financial restraints are an important factor to consider as people have lost jobs and savings, have had high medical expenses, or have seen daily spending increase through rising gas prices and the effects of inflation. In short, the world is not what it used to be.

The following are suggestions for ways to get involved with other people in some capacity, keeping in mind that we are all unique, that long Covid symptoms affect everyone in different ways, and that what works for someone else may not work for you. Many of my ideas are shaped by my patients' recommendations and experiences.

Social Engagement from Home

One of the silver linings of the pandemic is the way many companies and organizations shifted their business model to provide more online offerings, meaning it is now much easier to connect with the world without leaving home. If you are unsure about how to use technology, ask a family member, friend, or neighbor for a lesson. Some community organizations, libraries, and places of worship offer help with technology.

Communication with Family Members and Friends

- Texts: Great for checking in and shorter conversations.
- Group texts: A nice way for an extended family, for example, to post photos, share updates, and celebrate milestones.
- Phone calls: Especially helpful if they can be scheduled and consistent.
- Video calls: Many people prefer the intimacy of seeing someone's face or being able to catch up with several people at once, perhaps seeing children or pets in the background of a call. Scheduling a regular chat date allows you to prepare in advance.
- Social media: Facebook, Nextdoor, and other social networks can be a way to connect with others, perhaps keeping your network small to start and growing it over time. It is easy to add (or remove) people from your network of friends.
- Playing online games: You could play Scrabble, Words with Friends, Minecraft, Monopoly, or countless other games from your phone or computer with one or more players. Depending on what you choose, you can set up a time to play together or make your move independently and then wait for your opponent to make theirs.
- Enjoying an activity together: From watching a movie or TV show to other forms of entertainment, there are many options for social interaction without needing to leave the couch.

Reigniting Former Friendships

If you currently don't have people in your life to whom you can turn, an effective technique for making connections is to reach out to old friends and reengage dormant relationships that in the past have provided significant value. I'm thinking of people like neighbors on the street where you grew up, old teammates whom you've lost contact with but who continue to be important to you, long-lost friends from your wedding party, your second cousin's family. While they may not have been sitting by their phones for the last two decades waiting for your call, at least a few of them will be glad to hear from you and will be delighted to create space for you in their current lives.

In the early days of the pandemic, when we went into lockdown in Nashville, I decided to try this, reaching out to about twenty old high school classmates whom I had lost contact with over the years. After I heard back from a few, we set up monthly video calls where we reminisced about ball games, parties, various madcap antics, and the many changes we'd each undergone in the previous thirty-five years. This activity led to the formation of a small group text chat comprised of people whom I've known since my elementary school days. Now we text several times a week and sometimes daily, sharing pictures of the sun setting on the lake, sending birthday wishes, waxing nostalgic about summer camp, talking about the joys and challenges of adulting, and building each other up. The encouragement of these lifelong friends has become a surprising source of value to me and reviving such relationships may be worthwhile for you, too. Reminiscing about the good old days—far from a form of avoidance and denial—often provokes feelings of nostalgia, which research has consistently shown improves social bonds and self-esteem.

Other Online Options for Socializing

Possibilities abound for interaction with others—friends and strangers— via the internet. Some examples:

- Join a virtual movie night.
- Join a virtual book club—one popular place to do this is on Reddit, where there are thousands of communities devoted to virtually any topic.
- Play online video games—you can interact with anyone in a video game with a multiplayer platform.

- Interact in a work-sponsored virtual happy hour on Zoom or other platforms.
- Attend a meditation group or prayer meeting online each morning. One of my patients has joined a group and reports that it is incredibly empowering to pray with people from around the world every day.
- Take a class. There are many offerings online from cooking to financial literacy to yoga, some accessed free of charge via your community center, place of worship, or public library, while others will charge.
- Engage with social media. Many long haulers have found communities on different platforms, including Twitter, where an active contingent shares information, research, personal stories, and support about long Covid.

In-Person Socializing

- Meet-up groups. Through the website meetup.com, you can find new friends and join local communities based on hobbies, interests, or topics.
- Events at community centers and libraries. You may be surprised how many talks, classes, cultural events, and holiday celebrations take place at these institutions. They can be an excellent and low-key way to meet others.
- Volunteering. There are countless volunteer organizations looking for help and, depending on your interests, you'll likely find a meaningful and enjoyable role for yourself. Meet new people while doing good—which in turn will boost your own well-being.
- Places of worship. They often have thriving communities and frequent events and are welcoming to newcomers. Take a look at their calendar of services and/or talk to one of the leaders and let them know you're looking for social engagement and community. They will likely be happy to take you under their wing.
- Dog parks. With or without a dog, they are fun places to visit and

connect with local people. You'll find that dogs are great ice-breakers when it comes to conversations.

- Classes. Opportunities abound to join classes of all kinds, whether through educational institutions, cultural centers, or health and wellness centers.

WEAK TIES

If, despite your best efforts, you realize that creating intimate relational ties is challenging, the approach of cultivating "weak ties" may be better suited to you. The term hearkens back to one of the most definitive papers in the history of sociology, "The Strength of Weak Ties," by Stanford University professor Mark Granovetter, which demonstrated that well-being is not only influenced by a few close relationships but by casual interactions with many people—the security guard who says "Have a good evening!" whenever we leave the office for the day, the cheerful young adult who hands us our breakfast sandwich each morning at the fast food drive-through, or the pharmacist who always asks how we're doing when we call to refill a prescription.

I recently had an encounter with a weak tie—a seventy-five-year-old gentleman who was a few steps ahead of me in a 5K race for charity that I had decided to walk rather than run. During part of my stroll, we talked about the weather, the current state of politics, what it was like to send your kids to college, and the perils of the Vietnam War. I doubt I will ever see him again, but our small talk fostered in me a sense of belonging and connection and, as I left the city center, I felt grateful.

How to Cultivate Weak Ties

- Smiling at other people when you pass them on the sidewalk or at work, often sparking a conversation in the process.
- Check out at the grocery store using a cashier rather than a self-checkout option and begin to develop a personal connection. At our Kroger, I've developed relationships with Sonia, Bruce, and

Selvi. I don't know them well, but they've told me about their lives, and they've learned about mine, and we check on each other when we encounter each other multiple times a week.

- Initiate casual conversations with others whenever you have the opportunity, especially if you find that you and a new acquaintance have something in common. Many years ago, my wife and I were shopping at a store in Nashville, and I noticed a young woman wearing a University of Michigan sweatshirt. As a proud Michigander, this was all the encouragement I needed. I introduced myself, found that she and her husband had just moved to town from Ann Arbor, and invited them over to dinner. We didn't cultivate an active friendship, but we did cultivate a weak tie that I've maintained over the years on social media.

- If you have your groceries delivered or make most of your purchases online, make a plate of cookies for the delivery person. This will often spark a conversation.

- If you can't attend religious services in person, watch the service online, a popular option during the pandemic. Many virtual services allow people to participate in chats and some offer online discussion groups. You could consider engaging in a chat or group and, in so doing, developing a tie to this community.

- As a bonus, realize that in moments of serendipity, weak ties can become strong ties. Late last year, I was looking for a computer at my office to write a few notes, and I sat down next to a colleague whom I spoke to occasionally. As we stared at our screens, I initiated some small talk. It turned out that she loved hiking in Colorado and, like me, was a former college athlete (a much better one than me) and liked to read—we were the weakest of "weak" ties, but we obviously had much in common. A month or so later, we had a quick lunch, and this now-weekly lunch has been a fixture in my life for almost a year as we've moved from being barely acquaintances to close friends.

As you move through your days, I hope you notice your brief encounters with strangers and acquaintances, and perhaps can find ways to cultivate others in the hope that they may foster deep feelings of belonging and gratitude.

I've always loved poetry. I was inspired, I think, by my grandfather Earl Osterhout, a farmer from a pioneering family who wrote tender, sometimes witty verses that he thought of while plowing the fields and later transcribed on one of his prized possessions, a typewriter, occasionally publishing in the local paper. I'm not half the poet that he was but, if pressed, I can recite a poem or or two, having learned this skill in Asa Dawson's fifth grade class at Portage Central Elementary School. One of the poems I remember anxiously uttering in front of my class long ago has come to my mind a few times during the pandemic, namely "For Whom the Bell Tolls" by John Donne. Starting with the iconic words, "No man is an island / Entire of itself," it was written in 1624 but nearly four hundred years later it is as relevant as ever.

As you manage the effects of long Covid, you may feel isolated in many ways, but I hope that this chapter has encouraged you to find ways to spend time with others, to perhaps remind yourself of how good social contact can feel, and to realize that you have plenty to share with other people.

CHAPTER 9

BEYOND HEALTHCARE: Practical Help with Employment, School, and Disability

At a recent support group session, Teresa talked about attending her child's Little League baseball game, something she hadn't done in a while, as she found it too exhausting. Through tears, she said how thrilled her young son was that she was in the stands again but also sad because she hadn't been able to cheer for him after hitting his first home run. Like so many others with complications due to Covid, Teresa had vocal cord damage and could only speak in a raspy whisper. In a very literal sense, she had lost her voice.

As the conversation continued, I was struck by the fact that while Teresa's voice loss was real, many other long haulers experience a figurative loss of voice. Often limited by the fog of cognitive impairment and fatigue, burdened by feelings of shame and frustration around new life circumstances, and discouraged by a lack of answers from people in healthcare, they can find it hard to muster the energy to speak up for themselves. Often, they don't ask their doctors the questions that keep them up at night, presuming that they will be disbelieved, nor do they push back against disability insurance or workers' compensation decisions that may seem unfair or too complex and overwhelming to appeal.

Only now, a few years into the pandemic, are we beginning to comprehend the true impact of Covid and long Covid in virtually every area of life, from school to work to home—and to see the full extent of assistance that people need, in addition to medical treatment, to navigate and rebuild their lives. Even those with access to care for their long Covid symptoms still struggle to move forward, as the challenges and limitations of their illness rub up against the reality of schools, workplaces, and social settings. It is clear that long Covid is not only a health issue. I've seen patients withdraw from college when cognitive problems get in the way of coursework, or cling to jobs that they can no longer do, or forced into early retirement rather than be fired. Many have been let go. A recent *Washington Post* report estimates that up to 1.3 million long Covid patients are too sick to go back to work— they are left to grapple with the dire financial fallout, and mountains of paperwork if they are to stand a chance of receiving money from other sources.[1] These stories are repeated across a sweeping landscape of change affecting tens of millions of people in this country and around the world as they try to find and use the resources they need to get back on their feet.

In this chapter, I discuss concerns beyond healthcare that those with long Covid may have to navigate and provide practical ways for them to advocate for themselves. Over the years, I have helped patients obtain school and work accommodations, make return-to-work decisions, and gain financial support through disability insurance and workers' compensation, and I offer guidance and effective strategies here to ease the process.

MAKING RETURN-TO-WORK DECISIONS

For many people, long Covid interferes with their ability to return to work in the short or long term, and this sudden change in so central a part of their life can be devastating. For many of the patients I work with, their jobs, whatever they might be, are the bedrock of their financial stability and a core feature of their identity. In many instances, when they've been sidelined from work for a time, they are highly motivated to return and become, as they see it, productive again. Sometimes, however, this is easier said than done.

Some people may not be physically or psychologically ready to return to the job they held prior to getting sick, yet feel enormous pressure, whether financial, or from family members or themselves, to get back in the saddle. Sometimes the shame they feel at being away from work coupled with a desire to restore their lives to normal, as much as possible, can lead to hurried decisions and a rushed return—which can result in a cascade of outcomes such as termination, and financial and additional health problems.

For this reason, I always invite patients and support group members to engage in candid return-to-work conversations with their primary care physicians or other healthcare providers, and I am always happy to listen as they talk through their ideas and options. In some cases, even if they don't have clear opinions about the feasibility or appropriateness of returning to work, I can help create a framework to guide their thinking.

Points to Consider

- Why are you returning to work? Is this an absolute financial necessity or are other factors involved, such as anxiety, fear, or feelings of failure that you may associate with leaving the workforce?
- Is it realistic to return to work now? What are the nature and extent of your limitations?
- Will these limitations allow you to work in the same capacity as before or do you think you may need adjustments, perhaps in your schedule or in changes to your work environment or your duties? (I discuss these employer-provided accommodations in depth later in the chapter.)

- What about the need to attend doctors' appointments and follow-ups? Have you taken them into account?
- Would finding a less demanding job be a potential option? Or would you prefer to find a solution at your current job before pursuing this route?
- What are your health insurance options if you leave your job?
- Are there crucial reasons it might make sense to return to work for an abbreviated period, even if difficult—e.g., you are six months away from being fully vested, or from retirement, or you will be eligible for a large year-end bonus if you finish out the year?
- Is the stress or difficulty of returning to work greater than the financial burden of being without a job?
- If you cannot return to your job, are there other ways you can earn or receive money? Do you have a spouse or partner who works? What about disability insurance or unemployment benefits? Do you have any retirement savings?
- Have you assessed your financial situation accurately? Do you have more resources than you think, or do you have fewer? Would talking to a financial professional and/or accountant be a good idea?
- Do you need to return to the job you currently have or are there other jobs that may satisfy your financial, emotional, and family-related needs? How confident are you that you could get another job?
- How accurate are you in your evaluation of your strengths and weaknesses and your ability to succeed at a particular job? If you have cognitive impairment, how does that impinge on your judgment?

LONG COVID AS A DISABILITY

Peter, a long Covid survivor, is tall, thin, and in his early forties. He is a regional sales manager for a medical supply company, and has spent the last two decades crisscrossing the Southeast in a company car. After contracting Covid last year, a case that needed a telehealth appointment with his doctor but never a hospital visit, he developed persistent and profound fatigue. He took things easy for a few weeks and when his sick leave ran out, he returned to work. To his dismay, he realized that the twenty-mile commute to his office completely depleted his energy. He could barely get out of his car. How would he manage a full day's work? Or the two-hundred-mile drives to Memphis and beyond that were part of his sales route? He was scared he would lose his job, but he wasn't sure what he could do.

Fortunately for Peter and long haulers like him, in July 2021, the Biden administration announced that Americans experiencing long-term symptoms of Covid-19 might qualify for disability protections from the federal government if they "substantially limit one or more major life activities"—which might include walking, breathing, learning, or working.[2] The Office for Civil Rights of the Department of Health and Human Services and the Civil Rights Division of the Department of Justice went on to explain that long Covid can be a disability under federal laws that protect people from discrimination— Titles II (state and local government) and III (public accommodations) of the Americans with Disabilities Act (ADA), Section 504 of the Rehabilitation Act of 1973, and Section 1557 of the Patient Protection and Affordable Care Act.[3] In short, for long haulers like Peter, whose condition rises to the level of a disability, it can mean protections at work, school, and in the community, often in the form of accommodations or modifications.

ACCOMMODATIONS

An accommodation is a modification or adjustment to the way that things are usually done—whether at a job or in a work or school environment or a public setting—that ensures a person with a disability (defined as a mental or physical impairment that substantially limits major life activities or bodily functions) receives equal opportunities, so as to prevent discrimination against them.

Often my patients tell me the significant ways that their lives have been limited by long Covid, but when I talk with them about the possibility of applying for accommodations, they are surprised by the idea. Sometimes they are unfamiliar with the concept, or they may have heard the term but have not considered it relevant to their situation. However, if the effects of long Covid are getting in the way of carrying out day-to-day activities then it is likely that accommodations are applicable.

There are many situations in which long haulers may need to request accommodations and, while details will vary, the broad strokes of applying are similar.

Accommodations at Work

Qualified workers with long Covid have the right to accommodations if their symptoms are disabling as defined by the ADA, and the accommodation would not present an undue hardship to employers. Your employer must have fifteen employees or more for the law to apply. If your work is, or will be, impacted by your symptoms, there are several items to address before requesting accommodations:

Document the way your work is affected:

- Record your observations each day for several weeks.
- Some impacts may be obvious, such as energy or mobility limitations while others may be more subtle—maybe it is harder to concentrate when colleagues are talking nearby.
- Make a note of how your symptoms limit your work. Are you too exhausted to commute? Is your ability to stare at a computer screen lessened by cognitive impairment?
- If you have not yet returned to work, note symptoms as they apply in other areas of your life that are similar to your job duties.

This document will be useful for your doctor.

Think about changes that would make it possible for you to
carry out your job duties:

- It may be helpful to talk with others about this, such as family
  members or friends.
- Define the primary roles of your work and think about how you
  can still achieve them.
- Would it make a difference to work from home or telework? Or
  to take a short break every hour or so? Do you need flexibility to
  go to doctors' appointments?
- Be sure to think about potential objections from your employer
  and come up with arguments against them as well as alternatives
  that could more likely work in everyone's interest.

Be aware of common job accommodations provided under the ADA:

- Restructuring of the job and job tasks
- Physical changes to a workplace (installing a ramp or modifying
  a restroom)
- Modification of work schedules and allowing flexible schedules
- Reassignment to another position
- Modification of new equipment
- Installation of new equipment
- Providing qualified readers or interpreters
- Providing reserved parking
- Changing the presentation of tests and training materials
- Providing or adjusting a product, equipment, or software
- Modifying a policy to allow a service animal in a business setting

Speak with your healthcare provider about your work-related
limitations:

- Your employer may request documentation about your disability
  and/or need for accommodation if it is not known or obvious—
  but only as it relates to your request for accommodations.

- If you already have a doctor and/or healthcare practitioner treating your long Covid symptoms, set up an appointment to discuss specifically the ways your work is impacted. It can be most helpful to have one doctor (often your PCP) coordinate everything.
- Reach out to any specialists or other providers who have treated you and request records, labs, images, etc.
- Let your doctor know that you will be requesting accommodations and discuss potential options with them.
- Say that you will likely need a letter and documentation and ask if there is anything they will need from you to get this moving.
- If your struggles at work are the first indication that you might have long Covid, make an appointment with your PCP to discuss symptoms and their effects. Reading Chapter 1 again will be helpful to you.

Inform your employer that you would like to request accommodations:

- This is simply a request for a workplace change or adjustment because of a medical condition, impairment, or disability. It does not need to use specific language or to mention the ADA.
- It is best done in a meeting or phone call set up for the purpose, and while it is fine to ask for accommodations verbally, I recommend putting your request in writing, too, to make sure it is clear and to create a paper trail.
- Someone else, such as a spouse, coworker, or friend, can make the request on your behalf.
- Let your employer know that you have long Covid and the ways it limits your work.
- It can be best to follow your employer's lead and gauge their reaction, listen to their requests, questions, and ideas.
- After listening, suggest ideas for accommodations.
- Send an email after the meeting thanking your employer and

summarizing your request, their response, and what next steps are.

- Remember that you have the right to ask for reasonable accommodations and that it is usually in the company's best interest to keep you on as an employee, if possible.

Provide your employer with medical documentation:

- Your employer does not need documentation to provide accommodations but has the right to ask for it to understand how your work is affected by your disability.
- Don't worry if you don't have a long Covid diagnosis, as the aim of accommodations is to provide help for limitations caused by a disability, not for a particular condition.
- Ask your doctor to write a letter. It should be typed on their letterhead and include the nature and severity of your impairment, the activity or activities that it limits and to what extent, the requested accommodations, why they are needed, and how they will help.

Ideas for Accommodations Based on Long Covid Symptoms

Here are some accommodation ideas to explore for each limitation:

If you have shortness of breath with exertion, you could ask your employer to:

- Reduce physical exertion such as lifting, or standing.
- Use ergonomic tools to help with heavy lifting and exertion.
- Allow telework and/or flexible schedules.
- Allow regular breaks and rest periods.
- Allow time for medical treatment, such as use of a nebulizer or inhaler.
- Restructure work to remove unnecessary or secondary functions.

If you have extreme fatigue, you could ask your employer to:

- Allow regular breaks and rest periods.
- Provide an ergonomic workstation.
- Use ergonomic tools to help with heavy lifting and exertion.
- Allow telework and/or flexible schedules.
- Restructure work to remove unnecessary or secondary functions.

If you have anxiety and depression, you could ask your employer to:

- Allow telework and/or flexible schedules.
- Provide a modified break schedule and rest periods.
- Provide a quiet area/private space.
- Explore the possibility of allowing an emotional support animal at work.

If you have cognitive impairment, you could ask your employer to:

- Allow telework and/or flexible schedules.
- Provide a quiet workspace.
- Allow use of noise-cancellation or white-noise headphones.
- Provide uninterrupted work time.
- Provide a quiet, work-free zone for breaks.
- Provide memory aids, such as flowcharts and checklists.
- Allow regular breaks and rest periods.
- Restructure work to allow focus on essential job duties.

Peter, the medical supplies salesperson, became aware almost immediately on his return to work that he wasn't going to be able to perform his job as he used to pre-Covid. He arranged a telehealth appointment with his physician at the long Covid clinic and asked for advice. His doctor suggested that he pursue accommodations and offered to write a letter detailing the extent of his disability, should Peter's employer request one. "What is your main job requirement?" his physician asked. "Sales!" responded Peter. And that, he believed, he could still do whether he traveled across country or not. He was gregarious, engaging, and kindhearted, and the old-school Rolodex his dad had given him many years earlier Peter had filled to the brim with every key contact in a five-state area. All he needed was a computer with video conferencing.

Later that week, Peter met with his manager and gave a short presentation that he had practiced with his wife several times, one in which he described his situation, how his exhaustion limited his capacity to make in-person sales calls, suggested working from home or from the office, and explained how this would allow him to continue to meet the requirements of his job. When his employer asked for medical documentation, Peter was able to provide a letter from his doctor in which she cogently explained the basis of his fatigue and the ways that it impinged on his ability to drive long distances, and how his accommodations would overcome this. Eventually, Peter's request was granted. He was allowed to work from home approximately 80 percent of the time, with the remainder of his workdays spent either at the office or at a local sales appointment. It was a helpful and, to him, rather surprising outcome and allowed this high performer to remain in the workforce and keep on earning.

If things don't work out:

- Your employer must engage in an interactive dialogue about your request for reasonable accommodations. If you don't hear back, send an email to your employer and/or the head of human resources, requesting accommodations and why. Mention the ADA and that you have a legal right to a reasonable accommodation because of your disability.

- If you do not hear back after repeated attempts in writing to engage with your employer, it is time to turn to a disability lawyer. These can be found through a professional directory, but another good resource is your healthcare provider. They are often involved in supporting disability claims for their patients and may know disability attorneys. Many healthcare systems work closely with social workers, and they can assist you in finding an attorney as well.

- If your request is denied, your employer has no obligation to explain why, but they are often willing to do so.
- Denials can occur if an employer believes the requested accommodation(s) will cause them undue hardship, such as significant costs or disruption in the usual course of business. If this is the case, it may be appropriate to explore alternatives that could work for both parties.
- Depending on your employer, there may be processes or procedures to submit an appeal and, if so, you can pursue it.
- If your request is still denied, consult with a disability lawyer.

Accommodations at College

Accommodations are also available at both public and private colleges and universities for postsecondary students with disabilities, including those with long Covid symptoms that substantially limit one or more major life activities. On a college campus, accommodations are supports and services that help disabled students have equal access and opportunity to classes, programs, and student life. They can include academic accommodations, housing accommodations, or additional support, such as tutoring, and will be considered when they do not fundamentally alter the nature of a program, course, or service or present an undue financial or administrative burden.

As with employment accommodations, the onus is on the student to request accommodations rather than for the college to offer them, though once the request is made, many colleges are extremely helpful in guiding students through the necessary steps. In general, the process is similar to the one outlined earlier for employees with a disability, and I include a few higher-education-specific guidelines here:

Requesting accommodations:

- Everything will be handled through your college's Office of Disability Services (or Accessibility Services) and it is up to you to reach out to them. You can usually find information about the best way to contact them on their website.
- Usually, they will require information from you about your disability, how it impedes you in an educational setting, and what accommodations you need, and will ask you for current documentation.
- Look over the list of accommodations and services that they commonly provide and consider whether they might help you — and whether there are other modifications and/or supports that could be useful.

Documentation:

Each college or university has a formal process that varies slightly, but in general, students need a letter from a physician or mental health professional.

- Request a letter from your doctor or healthcare professional. If you have more than one overseeing your treatment, ask the person who is best equipped to speak to your specific struggles, understands the way they impact your daily college life, and is informed on ways that might help you to navigate challenges more easily.
- The more details you can provide to your doctor about your symptoms (type, severity, duration) with specific examples about how they play out — and limit you — in getting to class, taking notes, completing assignments, etc., the more easily your doctor can advocate on your behalf.
- Discuss with your doctor potential accommodations and how they can help your specific difficulties.

- Your educational institution will provide guidelines on documentation, but it is standard practice for your doctor's letter to cover the details of your disability and the way it limits your ability to function in an academic environment (with examples), to make specific accommodation requests and recommendations, and to explain clearly why they are needed.

Common student accommodations:

- Provide note-taking support including having a note-taker or the professor provide class notes if a student finds it difficult to take notes.
- Offer class attendance and deadline modifications. If a disability prevents a student from attending class or keeping up with coursework, professors can allow extra missed classes without penalties and can extend work deadlines.
- Provide extended time on exams and testing and/or a private or distraction-free testing room.
- Allow a reduced course load while still granting a student full-time status.
- Be flexible with seating arrangements; letting a student sit near the front of the class, for example.
- Provide assistive technology, such as recording pens and text-to-speech software.
- Offer sign language interpreting or transcribing in classes.
- Arrange for housing and dining accommodations, such as single or ground-floor rooms, flexible seating options in the dining hall, or the possibility of taking food back to the dorm.
- Allow a student to have a service animal or emotional support animal on campus.
- Provide disability parking, such as a reserved spot or the right to buy a long-term disability parking permit.
- Provide tutoring services (these are often available to all students).

If accommodations are granted:

- Let professors know that you have accommodations.
- Monitor the way the accommodations are working.
- Keep in contact with the Office of Disability Services in case adjustments are needed.

One of my patients, Wallis, told me she needed to drop out of college during one of our early sessions. "I'm failing my classes," she said. "I don't know what to do."

A freshman at a small liberal arts university in Tennessee, when she contracted Covid, she remembers feeling a bit "off" for a few days before developing the most profound feelings of fatigue she had ever experienced. She recalls falling asleep on the couch one Monday evening, draped in a blanket, watching the Dallas Cowboys, and waking up in a small room with her wrists in restraints and a breathing tube down her throat. This nightmarish experience continued for forty-six days until, as she puts it, she was spit out of the healthcare system on which she had come to depend. She found walking difficult and struggled with rudimentary cognitive tasks, but she desperately wanted to go back to college, a symbol of the old life she loved. Feeling optimistic, she took on a full load of course work but things didn't go as planned. Within weeks, due to her cognitive dysfunction, Wallis was failing three of her five classes and barely keeping up with the reading in the others. "I can't do it," she told me. "My brain doesn't work anymore. I'm going to quit and go home."

It soon became clear that she was not accessing the considerable resources at her disposal, partly because she didn't know about them but also because she found it very difficult to admit she had new deficits and limitations. To her, they conjured up feelings of failure and shame. Over time, I helped Wallis come to terms with the reality of her post-Covid changes, and we worked together to obtain accommodations through the Department of Student Services at her college.

In the letter I wrote, I described the specific problems her long Covid symptoms caused, including her limited ability to focus and her slower processing speed, which meant that note-taking was difficult and her work took longer to do. I proposed accommodations that would help to offset the impact of these problems, including more-flexible deadlines, use of a recording pen to take to classes to supplement her notes, extra time for tests and exams, and the possibility of taking proctored exams in a setting away from other students. With the benefit of accommodations—coupled with psychotherapeutic support—her academic performance improved, and she was able to get back on track with her classes and pass them all. She believes that with ongoing support this semester she will reach her goal and matriculate into the honors college.

If accommodations are denied:

- You will have the right to appeal a decision following a grievance procedure outlined by the college. Some colleges ask for more documentation, but many want to engage with the student in fully understanding the impacts of a medical condition or disability, so take the time to document and clarify as best you can.
- If your appeal is turned down, you can file an internal complaint with your school's 504/ADA coordinator if the school is a state-supported postsecondary school or any postsecondary school that receives federal funds.
- You may file a complaint with the Office for Civil Rights of the US Department of Education (OCR). More information about filing an OCR complaint is available on their website (ed.gov /about/offices/list/ocr).

WHEN ACCOMMODATIONS AREN'T ENOUGH

In many cases, as with Peter and Wallis, accommodations can be transformative and can help to keep someone in the workplace or in school;

however, sometimes they are not as helpful as people had hoped they would be. There are two primary reasons: 1) the needs of a particular job or program of study can make accommodations difficult to implement (for example, a sales job could be done at home but if the work involves showing new merchandise to vendors or demonstrating how new devices work, these accommodations may not be as helpful as they seem), and 2) the impairments you're experiencing might be so significant that even with well-crafted accommodations, the job or courses are too challenging (for example, if someone with PTSD has severe problems focusing, accommodations to reduce distractions may only help a little).

It can be difficult to view this outcome as anything other than failure, but it can be important to remember that it is one more step on a journey of finding out what works for you and what doesn't. In this scenario, what might happen next?

Resignation

If you're finding it hard to carry out your job requirements, even with accommodations, you may need to leave and transition out of the workforce or to a different job. In some cases, your employer may approach you to let you know they are going to have to let you go and give you a chance to resign, or you may decide to resign before this happens. There are theories on whether it is best to be fired or to resign, but this is not my area of expertise. However, if you choose to resign, it can be helpful to write a resignation letter. While it is not necessary, it is usually good practice. In a recent article in the *Harvard Business Review,* workplace expert Amy Gallo highlights three reasons it can be important: 1) it creates a paper trail, 2) it's customary in your industry or company, and 3) you feel like it will help manage the conversation.[4]

As with so many things, less is more in a good resignation letter. Keep yours short with details on why you are leaving, the date of your last day on the job, and a brief note of gratitude for the opportunities you've had. This may feel inauthentic and, if so, don't include it, but try to resist the urge to include angry, snarky, or petty comments, as they may and often do come back to haunt you. You may need a favorable reference from your current employer one day.

APPLYING FOR DISABILITY

If you have lost your job or are unable to work because you're grappling with the persistent effects of long Covid, you have likely turned (or will turn) to disability insurance, either private or public, for benefits. You may have found that it is not always easy to be approved and claims are often rejected.

Employee Plans

Private disability insurance is often offered by employers as part of an employee's benefit plan (about 40 percent of employers offer disability insurance and this option is especially common in larger corporations). Paid into over years, it is designed to be used in the event of someone developing an injury or illness that might prevent them from working—an illness like long Covid—with the insurance replacing part of an employee's income. Benefits are paid directly to the policy holder with no restrictions on how money is used. Sometimes benefits are short term, usually three to six months, while others are long term, with short-term policies paying more at once.

While specific claim information varies from policy to policy, the key hurdle is proving your disability, and I provide more information on this later in the chapter. In general, once a claim is filed, specific time frames are followed regarding decisions and, unless a special circumstance applies, you will be notified within forty-five days. If your claim is denied, you'll learn the reason why and have an opportunity to file an appeal, which will be evaluated by someone who wasn't involved in the initial decision. Again, you will be notified about the outcome within forty-five days. If your appeal is denied, it is fairly common to involve a disability law attorney to appeal again.

Social Security Disability Insurance (SSDI)

This federal program, paid for by workers and employees out of their payroll taxes, pays out monthly benefits in the event of a long-term disability that prevents someone from working for twelve months or more. If you have worked long enough, and recently enough, you would likely meet the non-medical requirements and could submit a claim via their website (ssa.gov/benefits/disability).

The general advice is to apply for SSDI as soon as possible, as the process is a lengthy one, often taking months for a decision to be made and many more months if an appeal is needed. It is imperative that your claim is detailed, accurate, and, crucially, meets the medical burden of proof that long Covid is substantially limiting one or more major life activities that are, in turn, preventing you from working. These could include walking, breathing, standing, sleeping, thinking, reading, leaving the house, or processing information, among many others. It is worth taking some time to get this right as the quality of medical evidence in your claim will play a significant role in whether it will be approved or denied. Nearly 70 percent of applications are denied the first time, often because of incomplete or inadequate medical evidence and documentation. There is also the challenge of having to prove that the illness is expected to last at least twelve months and, again, medical proof and documentation will be key.

Documentation for Disability Claims

In writing this section, I consulted with disability law attorneys whom I have worked with over the years. My aim is to help you in gathering evidence for your disability claim (whether for private insurance benefits or SSDI) but, obviously, I cannot guarantee that following this advice will result in your claim being approved, as everyone's circumstances are unique.

Supporting Documents

Your claim will need a detailed and supportive letter from your doctor or healthcare provider (more details below) as well as supporting medical documents.

- These include official notes and summaries from appointments, results from tests, imaging, etc.
- Save all medical documents in a safe place or request them prior to speaking with your doctor.
- Many healthcare systems have portals through which you can access medical records and, in some cases, print out notes, test results, and much of your health history.
- Inpatient medical records are also available, if needed, although depending on the length of a hospital stay, these can be challenging to wade through as they can be hundreds, even thousands of pages long. Often the single most helpful document is the discharge summary, which typically lists diagnoses made in the hospital as well as key details of the hospitalization, and a description of the course of the illness.

Choose Wisely Which Doctor to Ask

I've learned that patients have widely varying experiences with physicians when it comes to the ease with which they complete paperwork and the extent to which they provide advocacy. General practitioners and mental health providers are typically very willing to assist but patients often find it challenging to engage specialty providers.

Help Your Doctor Help You

- Have a candid conversation with your doctor about timelines and deadlines, and the urgency of paperwork as—speaking as a provider whose heart is in the right place—without such reminders it can be easy to forget.

- Ask for documentation/letters, etc., as far in advance as possible.
- Be organized.
- Send an email with a list of all your needs and deadlines, if possible, instead of multiple requests that may be harder for your doctor to follow.

The Supporting Letter

Healthcare providers vary widely regarding their experience in dealing with insurers as well as the Social Security Department. Some providers are seasoned and have written many letters on behalf of their patients while others may be new to the experience. In either case, it can be helpful to:

- Break your long Covid illness down into the symptoms that are most debilitating to your functioning. A letter that simply states that you have a diagnosis of long Covid is not likely to get your claim approved.
- Think carefully about what your job entails, how your disability impacts it, and make a list to share with your doctor.
- Highlight with your provider the details of your long Covid symptoms, the way they affect your functioning and inability to work, and connect them to objective medical evidence. For example, for cognitive dysfunction, objective evidence could include a neuropsychological test of executive functioning, or, for PTSD, details of an individual's responses on a structured clinical interview or PTSD assessment test.
- Show evidence of the way your disability prevents you from working. For example, if you are unable to stay focused in meetings, struggle to use technology, make frequent errors on key tasks at work, have problems meeting deadlines, and are unable to plan and organize complex projects, your doctor can elaborate that these cognitive deficits limit your ability to sustain focus on

specific tasks, transition easily from one task to another, multi-task, plan complicated projects, or devise efficient strategies to complete projects.

Current Medical Literature

I find it helpful to summarize in a paragraph or two relevant medical literature to provide context for the specific claims being made. This is especially important for long Covid, a relatively new illness (in terms of the history of medicine and disability claims) and not as familiar to adjudicators making disability decisions. There is compelling evidence documenting the many ways long Covid contributes to striking day-to-day challenges in many areas of functioning, but your PCP may need your assistance in locating it. A number of online repositories where long Covid advocates compile research are publicly accessible. Perhaps the most widely used repository is shorturl.at/irvX5.

Third-party Statements

- Have family members, friends, or coworkers write statements about the ways your functioning has changed since developing your disability.
- Statements should be detailed but specific and should clearly describe the ways that your functioning has been limited.

Using a Disability Lawyer, Representative, or Advocate

Many people pursue and receive disability without an attorney or advocate, and you may not need one. More frequently, people enlist their services when initial claims have been denied and, in this context, they can be extremely valuable. The cost of hiring a lawyer may be a concern, so it can be reassuring to know that Social Security disability attorneys don't charge upfront fees or require a retainer. Instead, they receive a contingency fee, only getting paid if you do. The Social Security Administration mandates that the total amount attorneys receive cannot exceed $6,000, though there may be small out-of-pocket expenses for you, too. The National Organization of Social Security Claimants' Representatives (800-431-2804) provides referrals for attorneys who specialize in disability determination through Social Security. The American Bar Association also has a referral service for disability lawyers by state.

Workers' Compensation

This state-mandated program (rules and regulations vary by state) provides compensation for medical expenses and treatments, and lost wages to employees who are injured (or even killed) in "the course and scope of the job." Many experts believe that contracting Covid while at work could fall under the rubric of workers' compensation benefits, so if you developed long Covid secondary to an on-the-job exposure, you may have a claim. This is especially true for certain employees including healthcare workers, first responders, and essential workers, and many states have extended workers' compensation benefits for these jobs. Consult your human resources department or an attorney if you have questions.

Many mornings, I take a hike on a trail a few minutes from my house. As I wind up hills, across flower-filled fields, and under the canopies of trees, I have an opportunity to reflect. One day, as I was walking, I found myself thinking about the way that many of the patients I've met since the beginning of the pandemic try to go it alone without asking for help. My thoughts were interrupted by a phone call from one of the very people I was thinking about. She was calling from a far-flung state more than a thousand miles away, crying as she related that she was ready to seek support. She had not wanted to before, she said, because she couldn't believe that she needed it. But it had made her path lonely, not easier.

Support can mean individual therapy or cognitive rehabilitation and, we have to remind ourselves, it can extend further into lives and include work and school accommodations or the decision to pursue disability benefits. In embracing support, patients can considerably improve their quality of life. Taking the step to consider these options can be humbling and hard but they are often worth considering with the help of your family and healthcare provider.

A FAMILY PROBLEM: Acknowledging Long Covid's Impact on Families and Healing New Fractures

When I developed OCD, I became consumed by the way my illness was affecting me, making me anxious, sometimes angry, turning me inward, and causing me to be preoccupied with my own needs. I wanted to imagine, and perhaps even pretended, that the challenges were mine alone, that I could fence them in, if you will, and that my family and friends could exist beyond the reach of the whirling vortex that threatened to engulf me. Of course, this didn't happen, and I had to admit that my illness, for better or worse, was their illness, too. This is usually the case—with mental illness, life-threatening illness, and chronic illness, including long Covid. And yet, for reasons that are unclear to me, the impact of long Covid on families receives less attention than it deserves.

I've seen this unfold in the media, both in the thousands of articles I've read and with the constant stream of reporters I've talked to. Many stories have been compellingly written or produced, brimming with scientific insights, thoughtful, and helpful, and yet their primary focus has been the persistent impact of Covid on the lives of patients and survivors—and not on the people they live with. Family members were forbidden access to their loved ones in ICUs and hospitals, especially during the first wave of infections, and when we did stop and think about how terrible this was, the narrative often highlighted the heartbreaking isolation of critically ill patients, without considering grieving and often terrified family members sitting in hospital parking lots or on the other end of a tenuous phone connection.

I'm not sure why this was and—to an extent—still is the situation. Perhaps it reflects the radical individualism so pervasive in the West or is a sign of the reductionist way we often think about illness, locating it "in" a person and forgetting the way it ripples out and impacts others. Whatever the case, it has made it appear, at times, that long Covid is an individual problem. There are probably millions of family members around the world who would beg to differ. This chapter offers guidance for those living with and caring for a family member with long Covid, including ways to focus on self-care and think about and discuss changes and challenges that may have arisen. I include suggestions for navigating conflicts, frameworks for effective communication, and advice on the often unique ways that distress is expressed by children, how to address it, and when to involve a professional.

THE IMPACT OF ILLNESS ON FAMILIES

Tommy slumped in the corner of a small medical office, his head in his hands. His wife, Georgia, was sitting a few feet away, crying, as she almost always did when conversations about Covid unfolded. The tension between them was palpable but it wasn't always this way. Married for fourteen years and parents of three children, they'd had their ups and downs like any couple but, for the most part, were a model of serenity and harmony until Tommy was fired from his job seven months earlier. Post-Covid cognitive impairment and shortness of breath had impeded his work as a senior air traffic controller at one of the busiest airports in North America and, while his employer had tried to find an alternative position for him, things hadn't worked out.

Now, Tommy spent his days at home, trying to catch up on household tasks, mending a leaky tap or cleaning out the garage; some days he would pick up the kids from school. He found it difficult. His identity had always been grounded in his role as a provider and now, without his job, he felt diminished. A heavy drinker a decade earlier, he had worked hard to quit with Georgia's support but recently he had started drinking again, a beer or two with lunch some days, a few more in front of the TV, and often a nightcap of half a bottle of Scotch.

Georgia was worn out with trying to keep her job while managing Tommy's doctor's appointments, their daughters' busy school schedules, and the thousand and one other things that needed her attention. Tommy was constantly irritable, even volatile, overreacting to his daughters, who had started walking on eggshells around him. One of them was struggling at school, another was on the precipice of an eating disorder, and the youngest had started wetting the bed. Georgia wasn't sure how long she could continue to handle everything.

It is not surprising that family members of long haulers often grapple with multiple challenges as they live with and care for their sick loved one and navigate the spillover effects of the illness in their own lives. In addition to daily caregiving tasks, worry about the illness itself, and what it may mean for the patient and the family now and into the future, there are often jarring changes to what psychologists call the family system, a way of functioning together that may have been in place for many years. Shifts in roles often emerge and new responsibilities are added as the need to focus on the illness and all that attends it supersedes everything else.

Unfortunately, old responsibilities are rarely subtracted, so someone who is already stretched to their breaking point with job demands, like Georgia, may have to make time and space to go to multiple doctors' appointments while singlehandedly ferrying children to soccer games and managing the household. Life can become a constant juggling act. Financial stresses often emerge, as even if families have high-quality health insurance, there can be significant other costs to bear in seeking out treatment, such as fuel, meals, sometimes lodging, and missed wages. And, as families try to adapt and adjust, multiple emotional and psychological reactions and responses often appear, adding complex layers to an already difficult situation.

While there is little if any research that focuses on the effects of long Covid on family members, there is much that we can extrapolate from other relevant studies. Investigations have long shown that chronic illness can cast a dark shadow in the lives of spouses, partners, and children, with mental health problems, including anxiety, depression, and PTSD, often emerging in family members.[1,2] A recent meta-analysis that reviewed the results of eighty-two investigations across twenty-five countries showed that in more than six thousand caregivers of people with cancer, primarily spouses, rates of depression were 25 percent,[3] and, in those caring for family members with other chronic health conditions, the rate was as high as over 70 percent.[4] Indeed, evidence consistently indicates that depression is more frequent in caregiving spouses than in the patients they care for.[5] Anxiety is also common, with some researchers asserting that it is even more prevalent in family members than depression. Studies also suggest that PTSD can commonly occur in families impacted by chronic illness, and in up to a third of family members following the critical illness of a loved one (including critical illness caused by Covid).[6]

Data consistently demonstrate that the spouses of chronically ill people report a lower quality of life than that reported by the chronically ill person, and that divorce rates are extraordinarily high in marriages in which one partner has a chronic illness.[7] One large study of almost three thousand married (different sex) couples, followed for twenty years, showed that 30 percent of the marriages ended in divorce.[8] Strikingly, divorce was more likely if the person with the chronic illness was a woman.[9] A recent study in the journal *Cancer* reports that in such cases, male–female marriages are six times more likely to end in divorce when the chronically ill spouse is a woman.[10] This finding is worthy of attention as, according to a study published in

Current Medical Research and Opinion, women are 22 percent more likely than men to develop long Covid.[11]

Challenges faced by families may include:

Taking Care of a Patient's Practical Medical Needs

Being a caregiver to someone with long Covid is a huge responsibility, demanding in time and often needing deep wells of emotional reserve. It may involve:

- Arranging and coordinating medical care
- Preparation for appointments
- Attending appointments and advocating for the patient
- Appointment follow-up
- Oversight of medications and refills
- Staying on top of new research and potential medical breakthroughs
- Filing insurance and/or disability claims

Physical Care

Depending on a loved one's symptoms, they may turn to you for physical support. This might include:

- Pushing them in a wheelchair
- Helping them navigate stairs or move around the home
- Helping them with aspects of daily living, such as getting dressed or in and out of the bathtub or shower

Taking on Additional Responsibilities

On top of caring for someone with long Covid, family members may take on tasks that may be too onerous for the patient:

- More shifts at work or juggling part-time or gig work to bring in extra income

- Handling budgeting and finances as money may be tight due to loss of income and additional medical expenses
- Grocery shopping and meal preparation
- Household management, such as paying bills and extra paperwork
- Taking on additional driving responsibilities
- Chores around the house and yard
- Children's needs including school, childcare, extracurricular activities, homework—and emotional needs, too

Changing Roles

These changes can take place in subtle ways over time:

- Caregiver/care receiver roles can become entrenched and take over marriage or partnership roles
- A greater focus on the illness may mean less focus on relationships
- Family hierarchy may change, which can bring stress and resentment
- More dependence on a family member can mean less independence for a patient in detrimental ways
- Children may have to grow up quickly to take on new responsibilities

Navigating Life Changes Beyond the Home

When caring for someone, the illness can become central, with everything else orbiting around it, and life can become narrower than it once was.

- Life becomes more homebound due to physical, emotional, and financial barriers
- There is less time for relationships with others
- Socializing becomes limited

- There may be concerns about what others think or that they won't understand
- Trips beyond the home are illness-focused and practical (appointments, grocery shopping, picking up prescriptions) rather than for pleasure or relaxation

Helping to Manage a Patient's Emotions

Sometimes patients struggle with their emotions about being sick, and this can impact family members.

- Partners and children can be on the receiving end of many emotions, such as anger, sadness, hopelessness, and frustration.
- There may be the need to manage the patient's perceived feelings of being a burden and validating their struggles.
- Patients may need to talk, so it can be helpful if family members are willing to listen.
- Sometimes substance use can occur, which brings its own difficulties for loved ones to contend with.

Changes in Your Emotional Well-being

It's natural for family members to feel a wide range of emotions while caring for a loved one struggling with long Covid. These may include:

- Sadness for the family member and for the changes in your own life
- Anxiety brought on by life stressors
- Fear that your loved one may never get better, or may get worse
- Frustration about the ongoing situation
- Anger—at the illness, society's response to the pandemic, your family member, or that your life has changed so drastically
- Guilt about feeling sad and frustrated when you are not suffering from an illness

- Lack of motivation because there doesn't seem to be any point to anything

Changes in Your Physical Well-being

A new and uncertain life situation and the demands of caregiving can bring on physical symptoms or may lead to behaviors that can impact health:

- Exhaustion due to the sheer number of responsibilities/activities crammed into each day, or lack of restful sleep
- Sleep problems, such as difficulties falling asleep, staying asleep, or waking early
- Unhealthy eating, such as fast food as it's quick to prepare and comforting after long days
- Alcohol or drug use as a way to relax and feel distance from the reality of life

Helping Children Navigate the New Normal

For families with children, there are often additional changes and stresses that can arise. These may include practical elements—the logistics of childcare, school needs, and extracurricular schedules—but may also involve a child's emotional response to a parent's (or other family member's) illness on a day-to-day level as well as on an existential one. Later in the chapter, I provide more detailed guidance on helping children cope and thrive when a family member, especially a parent, has long Covid.

THE VORTEX OF LONG COVID

The unfortunate reality is that living with long Covid will impact the patient's life in multiple ways, and their family is likely to be caught up in the vortex of illness, too. Difficult as it may be, it can be helpful to acknowledge this as fact, to pledge to address it together, and to try and minimize potential damage by using the following strategies: self-care for the caregiver, effective and open communication, and freely expressing emotions (even the negative ones).

Coping by Focusing on Self-Care

Many years ago, at the VA hospital, I saw a patient, Jeremiah, for a PTSD evaluation. He was thoughtful, gentle, altruistic—and profoundly traumatized. He told me he'd been sitting at a bar on a river in Wisconsin, enjoying a Saturday night beer with friends, when he saw a woman behind the wheel of an old wood-paneled station wagon speeding down a boat ramp into deep water. He realized she was trying to kill herself. Jeremiah wasn't a particularly strong swimmer and, as a former infantryman, he had spent more time in the desert than in the water, but he rose from his table, took off his steel-toed work boots, and dove into the river, determined to save her. He managed to pull the woman from the car without much difficulty, but as he started to swim to shore with her in tow, she began to panic and flail. She no longer wanted to die, and, using Jeremiah as a ladder, she tried to save herself from the depths, clambering over him and pushing him down. There is a lot about that evening that Jeremiah doesn't remember but his words to her, as they battled in the water, have always stuck in his mind: "Lady, if I drown, I won't be able to help you get to shore."

I've thought about this story many times since Jeremiah first told me and I've seen it take on many different forms. It's expressed by airline attendants who remind travelers that if oxygen masks deploy, they should don their own masks first and then go about the business of helping others, and by therapists who tell troubled couples that a good way to support their child with behavioral problems is to work on fixing their marriage first. I've long appreciated the wisdom of the viewpoint that you are better able to help others when you take care of yourself, and I've seen it at work again and again in recent years in the lives of family members living with and caring for long Covid patients.

Here and on the pages that follow I highlight practical ways to cope, recognizing that as you bolster your mental health and build resilience by caring for yourself, you'll be better equipped to handle the many challenges before you.

- *Talking it out:* In general, this is the opposite of internalizing, which refers to pushing thoughts and feelings down. Later in the chapter, I'll address ways to have conversations with your ill family member, but here talking is for you—to be heard, seen, and recognized for all the hard things you are facing and dealing with, for how your life has changed.

- *Talking with a therapist or social worker:* If anxiety or depression is getting in the way of your daily functioning, I advise speaking with a professional. But even if you don't think you reach the criteria for a mental health condition, and you have time, energy, and resources, you may find regular appointments an invaluable support. If in-person resources are hard to find, a variety of apps exist for connecting with a therapist online. Some good options are summarized in a recent article on Verywell Mind (verywell mind.com/best-online-therapy-4691206).

- *Support groups:* They do exist for family members of long haulers (see Chapter 8 for finding support groups in general) or you may find one for family members of the chronically ill—they can be helpful in providing fellowship and advice, for feeling less alone on your journey.

- *Talking with a friend:* Something formal may not seem right for you and you may prefer to chat with a friend or relative. If so, try to make it a habit. Making contact and talking with someone outside your usual day-to-day life can be enormously helpful.

- *Asking for specific help:* Even the most well-meaning people don't think about the toll that caregiving can take, and you may need to ask for help with certain tasks such as childcare, carpooling, dog walking, transportation, and grocery shopping. You're likely to find, though, that when you ask, people are more than happy to offer assistance, especially if you define a specific task or role for them. And if someone does volunteer to help without being prompted, accept immediately. If you can, when you delegate a task or two try to use the time and energy gained on self-care.

- *Exercise:* The benefits of exercise are well documented for both psychological and physical health and include improvements in mood, concentration, sleep, and productivity as well as lowering blood pressure and boosting good cholesterol levels. Exercise can be a helpful way to relieve tension and get away from the incessant demands of life. For some, it may mean an intense workout at a gym but there are many other forms of exercise that are broadly available to almost everyone—strolling in the park or your neighborhood; walking up and down stairs during your lunch break at work; joining an outdoor workout group (these have sprung up around the world since the beginning of the pandemic); strength training at home with simple tools like a medicine ball, dumbbells, or a set of resistance bands; yoga (perhaps taking an online class) for various skill levels, including chair yoga, and simple stretching.

- *Engage with nature:* Not very long ago, wild and natural spaces were the domain of hunters, fishermen, and outdoor enthusiasts but over the last two decades there has been an explosion of research interest in the benefits of nature for everyone: dog walkers, urban gardeners, retirees, and others who may never climb Mount Kilimanjaro but love to roam through nearby woods, sit in the backyard watching hummingbirds, or spot frogs at their local park. In one large British study conducted at the University of Exeter, researchers studied nearly twenty thousand people and found that spending two hours or more each week immersed in nature was associated with substantially better overall health and psychological well-being.[12]

To weave nature time into your week, go for a short walk close to home, near trees or a park if possible. Buy a houseplant or two to care for indoors, or a few herbs to start an herb garden. Bird-watch through a window. Seek out gardens, parks, or wild spaces as you go to appointments or carry out errands, and try to stop for a few minutes and admire them from the car or from outside.

- *Sleep:* Recently, I met with one of my patients at the ICU Recovery Center to continue our informal investigation into his behaviors, trying to figure out an underlying connection to the fairly frequent conflicts he had with other people. As we talked, it became clear that his angry outbursts and relational dust-ups usually followed an evening of very poor sleep. His story is like mine and may be like yours. Sleep is often the tail that wags the dog and influences how we behave while powerfully shaping our ability to cope with stress.

  While it may seem as if there are not enough hours in a day to accomplish everything you need, taking small steps to improve sleep can make a dramatic difference. The first step is to prioritize sleep. Add it to the to-do list, give yourself a set bedtime, and aim to check it off each day. Try to have a simple wind-down routine for an hour before sleep, nothing fancy; for instance, no eating or alcohol during that hour, limited screen time, and engagement in stress-free activities. Other tips include writing your worries down and assigning them a specific timeslot in the coming days to address them, reducing your caffeine intake, going to sleep and waking up at the same time every day, and limiting daytime naps.

- *Meditation:* This widely used mental practice can help you calm your body and mind, center yourself, and relax in the midst of the frantic rush of life. When carried out on a regular basis, it can also improve immunity and physical health and relieve pain and fatigue. Meditation classes are available in person and online, but many people have found meditation and brought it into their lives through various popular apps. Several patients have mentioned Headspace, Insight Timer, and Calm as their go-to for guided meditations, but a quick online search will provide you with many different options to find one that might work for you. Once you have learned the basics, you'll be able to meditate virtually anywhere—while working out, making the bed, watering the flowers, or taking a train.

- *Breathing exercises:* Deep breathing allows you to move more air into your body and, as a result, can create a calming effect, reducing anxiety and stress. It has been shown to improve psychological well-being, decrease stress, reduce high blood pressure, and help with falling asleep. One simple technique is triangle breathing, in which you slowly breathe in through your mouth (four seconds), let your belly fully expand (four seconds) and breathe out through your nose (four seconds).

- *Engage in a hobby:* In the pressure cooker of life with a chronically ill person, hobbies may seem unimportant, a frivolity in the face of serious matters, and that is precisely why I would encourage you to continue with, or begin, one, with the goal being that these pursuits can promote self-care. Perhaps you enjoy baking bread, crossword puzzles, skateboarding, or singing in a choir. Or maybe you've always wanted to learn another language. Try to give yourself a few minutes a day, several times a week to pursue a passion and reconnect with a sense of fun, of purpose, away from thinking about long Covid for a while.

I'm not much of a cook but I love to smoke barbeque and, during the first year of the pandemic, when many of us were confined to our homes, I decided to try and build my own smoker, hoping it would be a buffer against the stress I was feeling. My longtime dream was a handsome smoker made from a whiskey barrel, gleaming with shiny knobs and thermometers, and capable of creating a delicious family meal. With this in mind, I bought an old barrel, some ancient power tools, and settled down to work, happy to have a hobby I could turn to now and then at the end of a long day or on weekends. In just a few months, I had created my vision.

One June morning I prepared a turkey, filled the newly made smoker with lump charcoal, then, with happy anticipation, lit it on fire. About fifteen minutes later, during a Zoom call, I watched the entire smoker erupt in flames, leaving behind nothing but ashes. I was disappointed, to say the least, but I learned something important that day—that the process of engaging in a hobby is perhaps even more important than the outcome, because it is the thing that gives you joy.

- *Music:* Listening to, playing, and singing along to music has been shown to significantly reduce stress through different mechanisms, including by decreasing heart rate and cortisol levels and by releasing endorphins.[13] It can also reduce pain. Whatever genre you enjoy the most is the one to play.

Coping by Effective Communication

Recently, I sat down with a lovely couple in the ICU Recovery Center for a therapy appointment. The wife was recovering from a case of Covid that had nearly killed her and was still having difficulties many months later. As we were talking, her husband said that her persistent symptoms of long Covid were the elephant in the room, something that they both tacitly acknowledged but resisted talking about. "I don't want to burden her with it," he said. "Not after everything she's gone through...is still going through." He suggested quietly that the elephant could no longer be ignored but if they discussed it, his wife would cry, he would cry, and they would be overcome with difficult emotions. My response to him? "Exactly."

This was precisely the process I wanted them to engage in—to be open and honest with each other, even if it provoked unpleasant feelings, because such vulnerability promotes connection and intimacy. They would be crying, yes...but they would be crying together. I wanted them to talk about what life with long Covid meant to each of them, to their relationship, and how they could best get through it together. I hoped we could lay the groundwork for effective communication.

Many family members hide their thoughts and feelings about their experience with their loved one's illness, perhaps believing they don't have permission to unburden themselves, or to have their own needs, so they suffer in silence. This isn't helpful to anyone in the long run as it can lead to burnout and resentment, which, in turn, can fracture relationships.

When patients and their families choose connection over avoidance, isolation, and self-protection, it builds a foundation from which difficult things can be navigated together. Being truthful without imposing on another person can sometimes feel like a delicate dance, and effective communication is key. Here and on the following pages are strategies for speaking honestly in a way that neither judges nor blames but instead promotes the well-being of everyone in the family.

- *Schedule a time to talk:* It can be helpful to schedule talks or discussions ahead of time so that no one is caught off guard. It doesn't have to be formal, just a simple phrase such as, "I have a few things I'd like to talk through with you. Can we find time after lunch?" In this way, you can be sure that a discussion doesn't start with heightened emotions or at a time when your sick family member is exhausted. Be flexible and willing to change the time as necessary.
- *Embrace — or at least allow for — uncomfortable emotions:* Feelings of grief, loss, and, often, anger can bubble up as couples and families engage each other in conversations about how they feel. You may prefer to suppress these so-called negative emotions, or not to witness them, but that won't make them go away. Let each other talk, even about your darkest emotions, and try not to shut these conversations down, even if it seems tempting. You don't need to

find solutions. Instead, expressing emotions, talking, listening, and showing empathy are most important here. By sitting with uncomfortable emotions together, you create deep bonds that can carry you through these difficult times.

- *Take a break:* If, after a while, it gets too uncomfortable, you can take a break. Try saying, "I really want to talk about this but I'm finding it hard. Can we talk again tomorrow morning?" And then, of course, you have to commit to having another conversation the next day.

- *Strive to prioritize the right things:* You may have no idea what to say or what solutions to offer. That's okay. More important is your affirmation that you'll be a steady, reliable presence while trying to figure things out, that you're on this journey together, wherever the road winds.

- *Advocate for yourself:* If you are feeling overwhelmed or discouraged, speak up. Use words that explain and don't blame. Make "I" statements that emphasize how you feel but embed them in compassionate language. For example: "I'm exhausted by everything right now, the caregiving, the kids, and I know it's not your fault or theirs. But sometimes I need to say it out loud and have someone say, 'Yes, it's hard.' " Say when you need to take a break. While you may be angry or frustrated or feeling as if you might explode, try to use language that explains without getting too emotional, such as "I'm feeling stressed. I'm going to walk to the store to clear my head and then I'll be back."

- *Try not to take things personally:* When dealing with the challenge of chronic illness, it's inevitable that unkind words are said, even when families are trying their best. Try to recognize that sometimes people say things that they don't mean and act in ways that are not compatible with their values. If you have said something that you now regret, be quick to apologize. "I'm sorry I said that. I really didn't mean it, and I'm sorry I upset you." If you have been on the receiving end, try to give the benefit of the doubt. If you find that there is a lot of animosity heading in your direction or that you are often angry and lashing out, it's time to have a conversation. "I've noticed that you seem to be angry with me a lot of the time and it's hard for me to take. Can we figure this out?"

- *Remember, understanding must precede advice:* This insight is the brainchild of marriage and family therapy luminary Dr. John Gottman. Much of the time, when we see family members hurting, we're quick to try to fix the problem, but this approach, while natural, is usually unhelpful. Instead, ask questions and seek to understand, displaying empathy in the process, before engaging in the hard work of shared problem-solving.

- *Focus on the relationship:* While talking and being open about the impacts of illness is good, it is equally important to spend time *not* talking about it. Aim to spend time together as you used to before illness entered your lives and/or find new ways to engage. These can be active or passive—you could plant tomatoes in a garden together or hold hands while sitting on the porch. What matters is participating with each other in a shared experience and continuing to build bonds.

  Michelle and I have learned to do this, especially when my illness rears its head, and while togetherness can potentially take elaborate forms, I'm learning that simple rituals are often the most powerful—walks in the neighborhood, time spent cooking and enjoying a meal, discovering a new TV series to binge watch, or simply going to the store together. One of my patients looks forward to twice-weekly phone calls with her cousins, something they used to do years ago and have resumed now that she is homebound so much of the time.

- *Remember you're not mad at each other but at the situation:* Nerves fray and tempers flare, and anger, particularly if expressed in unhelpful ways (e.g., rage, resentment, passive-aggressive behavior) can get an unhealthy foothold in a relationship. When these feelings emerge, have the courage to pause and look beneath the surface to see what emotions may be underlying them—perhaps sadness, fear, or disappointment—and try to process them. The fury you may feel when your adult daughter loses the car keys again may really be a sign that you're scared that her cognitive dysfunction is getting worse. Recognizing that other emotions may be involved can help you direct your feelings away from your family member. If you're going to be angry, be so at the situation—as a team—more than you are angry at each other.

- *Seek professional help:* If, despite your best efforts, effective communication eludes you or breaks down, consider working with a therapist or counselor. In particular, marriage and family therapists are trained to work with couples. It can be helpful to have a neutral and experienced voice in the room to guide the conversation and navigate thorny issues.

HELPING CHILDREN COPE

A few months ago, I received a phone call from a woman in South Carolina named Lily who reached out to me after reading an article about our work with long Covid patients and their families. In her mid-forties, she was warm and thoughtful, and after we established a quick and easy rapport, she told me her story—a tale of a close-knit family, a teenage daughter, a husband who had been a director of operations at a large construction firm, and the challenges they'd endured over the previous year.

Her husband, Gilbert, developed Covid and spent seventy-four days in the ICU, then twenty more in the hospital, before transitioning to a rehabilitation center and eventually home. During much of his critical illness, they hadn't known if he would survive and, on two occasions, a priest was called to his room to perform last rites. Now, he was doing better though some symptoms lingered and he was often short of breath and needed supplemental oxygen. He had returned to work in a limited capacity at a different job—one with considerably less pay, but with fewer demands to accommodate his health struggles.

Lily, on the other hand, had taken on extra work as more of the financial responsibility shifted to her, and while she loved her job, there were downstream effects. She was less present at home and less emotionally available and, as time passed, their daughter, Olivia—usually a lively, effusive teen—began to struggle. Normally a good student, she had just earned a *D* on a calculus midterm. She was confrontational with Lily, angry that she was "never home and didn't care," and "that Dad was always too tired to do anything," and she was starting to spend most of her time in her room. One evening, when she couldn't reach her father on the phone, she had a panic attack and was almost inconsolable until he pulled into the driveway.

Lily wondered if her daughter might be grappling with trauma due to her father's illness and his ongoing health struggles with long Covid. While I'm always disinclined to give medical opinions over the phone, I privately thought so, too, and agreed with Lily's idea to seek a formal consultation. A little while later, I learned that Olivia had seen a psychologist and started cognitive processing therapy for PTSD.

Mental health difficulties are common in children, adolescents, and emerging adults, and rates of anxiety and depression have almost doubled during the pandemic. In an influential meta-analysis in *JAMA Pediatrics* in 2021, authors reviewed twenty-nine different studies of more than eighty thousand children (all eighteen years old or under) from across Central and South America, East Asia, Europe, the Middle East, and North America, and documented rates of anxiety of 20.5 percent and depression of 25.2 percent—compared with rates of anxiety and depression in children of 11.6 percent and 12.9 percent, respectively, before the pandemic.[14]

While little data is available on the prevalence of mental health disorders in children of long Covid patients, data from other roughly analogous populations may be a reliable guide. Investigators have consistently found that the children of people with chronic illness frequently struggle with psychosocial adjustment and, in particular, are often more likely to internalize problems,[15] developing issues with anxiety[16] as well as somatic symptoms.[17] Research shows that children and adolescents living in a household where a family member has a chronic illness are at greater risk for mental health difficulties than children living in a household where no family member has an illness.[18] This increases if the sick family member is a parent. One large Australian study of more than nineteen thousand kindergarteners demonstrated that difficulties in areas including emotional health, language development, and communication can begin at a very young age in children of chronically ill parents.[19] In the case of college students, research has shown the presence of more anxiety, stress, and depression in those with chronically ill parents than those without.[20]

It can be extremely hard for children and adolescents to cope with a family member's illness, especially if it is the parent or parent figure who is ill, and to navigate the ways, large and small, that it impacts their lives. They may worry that a parent with long Covid may never get better or may die, or they could feel angry that their parent can't play soccer or lift them up for hugs anymore. They may overhear conversations about financial concerns and absorb the stress, or they may sense discord and an atmosphere of uncertainty and secrets and become scared by not knowing. Their reactions may manifest in many different forms, some more overt, as Olivia's were, such as declining school performance, sadness, and isolation, or in behavioral changes such as bedwetting and temper tantrums, or in striving to be the perfect child so as not to cause their parents more worry.

There are strategies to help children and young adults face and handle difficult situations and navigate the challenge of having a family member struggling with long Covid, including honest conversations, permission to express their feelings, and tools for handling emotions.

Having a Truthful Conversation

While some parents worry that telling the truth about a difficult situation may increase a young person's anxiety, I have found the opposite is true.

- Find a good time to sit down and tell your child what is going on at home, the medical struggles and how they may unfold. This may include saying that Mom has a sickness and that she's getting help or trying to get help from doctors and nurses, or that Dad's brain doesn't work in the same ways as before and he has left his job to focus on getting better.

- Use age-appropriate language and details while making sure you are telling the truth.
- Ask your child if they have questions and let them know that their questions are welcome, even if they may make you sad.
- Be honest about how you're feeling. You may say, "It makes me sad that Mommy is not well." Let your child know how you cope with sadness, for instance, "Dad likes drinking hot chocolate, and making him some makes me happy" or "Sometimes I go for a run and that can make me feel better."
- Children may ask difficult questions, such as whether a parent may die. Answer honestly that it is unlikely while also reassuring your child that there will always be people to look after them, no matter what.
- Acknowledge that changes to the family system have developed that make things different and hard while stating that you are still a family and will get through this together.

Expressing Emotions

- It may seem too much to bear when your child expresses anger or sadness that their parent can't do certain activities anymore, or that there isn't as much money for special treats. But let them feel those emotions and help them know that "negative" emotions are appropriate for what they're going through.
- Don't shame or berate them for their feelings. Don't say, "How could you say that? It's not your uncle's fault!" Instead agree with them that it is sad, or frustrating, and help them find ways to manage their emotions (suggestions on the next two pages) or find alternatives. "I can't go in the kiddie pool with you, but I can watch you from here!"

- If your child is happy, giggling, and having fun, and seems oblivious to what you may be going through, accept that it may be their way of dealing with the situation, of dosing their sadness.
- If older kids seem moody and want to be anywhere but home, allow them some freedom to be with friends or engrossed in activities that have nothing to do with long Covid. Just let them know they are missed when they are out of the house and try to have certain evenings or times set aside for family time, whether eating meals together, having movie night, etc.

Managing Emotions

As mentioned, help your child know that they may feel lots of different emotions, that all their feelings are natural, and that they can get through them by using different tools such as:

- Listening to or playing music
- Singing songs
- Playing sports
- Writing in a journal
- Making art
- Seeing a friend
- Looking at or reading books
- Engaging with a pet
- Cuddling with a soft toy
- Talking on the phone or texting with friends or family
- Going for a walk
- Deep breathing

EMOTIONAL AND BEHAVIORAL RESPONSES

It is to be expected that children will have emotional and behavioral responses to the upheaval and unexpected shifts in their lives brought on by long Covid, especially when experienced in tandem with difficult and far-reaching impacts of the pandemic. However, it's important to be aware that a child's behaviors could signal the presence of a mental health condition that may need to be monitored by watchful waiting or may benefit from further intervention. I list symptoms below that are associated with anxiety, depression, PTSD, and eating disorders in order to educate rather than alarm.

Anxiety

- Separation anxiety — e.g., extreme or exaggerated fear of being away from a loved one (usually a parent)
- Developing new and increasingly severe worries — either general or very specific
- Being afraid of social situations, leading to anxiety about attending school, or many other places
- Changes in sleep — may have nightmares, and may not want to sleep alone
- Signs and symptoms of panic — often physiologic symptoms like sweating or a racing heart
- An increase in somatic complaints, such as stomachache, headache, lack of appetite, tense muscles, or exhaustion
- Concerns that a parent may die or that they may never get better
- Heads to the school nurse's office more frequently than usual

Depression

- Withdrawal from relationships or from previously enjoyable activities
- Increased irritability
- Significant changes in academic or athletic performance
- Inability to concentrate
- Spends a lot of time watching TV or playing computer games
- May lack the energy or inclination to do anything at all

- Changes in appetite
- Self-destructive behavior—e.g., cutting

PTSD

- Re-experiencing the event (or series of events)—e.g., a parent being in the ICU with Covid-19
- Avoidance of trauma—refusing to talk about it and becoming emotional when others do, such as leaving the dinner table when family members are discussing the parent's long struggle with Covid-19
- Nightmares
- Being constantly on edge, especially as it relates to concerns about a parent's physical symptoms
- Anger, irritability, and, especially, reactivity
- Social withdrawal

Eating Disorder

- Marked changes in weight
- Excessive exercise
- Preoccupation with nutritional content and information (a focus on calories)
- Obsessive concern about body image
- Use of laxatives or related over-the-counter products
- Rigid rituals around food
- Skipping meals
- Wearing layers or oversized clothing

WHEN TO BE CONCERNED

Mental health conditions exist on a spectrum that ranges from behaviors that are slightly different from normal functioning to behaviors that are clearly atypical and, ultimately, could be harmful. It is often difficult for parents to decide if or when a child's symptoms require evaluation or treatment by a professional, especially as some ups and downs are likely, just as they are for adults, when undergoing life changes. But there is a time when it's appropriate to help your child by reaching out for formal mental health support. Here are some guidelines:

- *Symptoms last for a long time:* Issues with worry or sadness typically abate quickly after they first emerge, often within a week or two, so if significant symptoms persist for more than a few weeks, consider seeking professional help. If the stressor that plays a role in causing symptoms persists (e.g., Mom not being able to get off the couch or struggling to read bedtime stories), as it often does with long Covid, symptoms may persist as well. In this case, consider the other guidelines offered here, too.

- *Symptoms interfere with functioning:* Mental health symptoms may be mild and, though present, may not interfere with everyday functioning. However, it is time to seek out an evaluation if your child or young adult finds it hard to consistently carry out their usual tasks, responsibilities, and social activities. This might include difficulties at school or school refusal, getting fired from a cherished weekend job, or unexpected conflicts with their high school track coach.

- *Symptoms raise concerns about safety:* Seek treatment immediately if symptoms include self-harm. This may take the form of explicit comments about suicide or vague comments about wanting to die, or not wanting to be around anymore. Cutting, usually carried out with razor blades, knives, and pieces of glass, is also a concern and often a sign of significant distress. Self-harm can be hard for parents to understand or accept, but it is not something to ignore in the hopes that it will go away.

- *Symptoms indicate an eating disorder:* Eating disorders (ED) such as anorexia nervosa and bulimia nervosa are potentially life-threatening conditions that affect people's emotional and physical health, and symptoms should be taken very seriously. They are distinct from conditions like anxiety and depression, but many people with anorexia nervosa, in particular, battle both. Rates of inpatient hospitalizations for adolescents with eating disorders have doubled during the pandemic, though the prevalence of ED in children of long haulers is unknown. It's important to know that eating disorders are not a lifestyle choice or a fad, and that a supportive family can be key in helping someone to get help. If you notice red flags, please have a conversation with your doctor or your pediatrician.

HAVING A CONVERSATION

Recognizing the presence of likely problems is an important first step that needs to be followed by a conversation with your child or young adult. Not surprisingly, it is a conversation you may be reluctant to have, perhaps because you are unsure how to begin or worry you will make things worse. Remembering that perfect is the enemy of good, make a commitment to talk to your child, recognizing that what you say may make less of an impact than the love, empathy, and understanding you show.

- Find a good time to talk when you can focus on the conversation.
- Talk openly about your concerns and use specific examples. ("I've noticed that you've stopped hanging out with your friends and spend a lot of time alone in your room.")
- Be as explicit as you want to be. If you are concerned about the possibility of suicide, say so. Don't use euphemisms or beat around the bush. ("I've heard you saying that you wish you were dead, and I'm concerned you're thinking about suicide.")
- Use positive body language (open hands with palms up, arms uncrossed, eye contact) and don't be defensive to the feedback you will likely receive—whether it is given in a whisper or a shout.

- Talk about your own struggles, if appropriate, as a way of normalizing their experience. ("I've been feeling angry that this is happening to our family, too.")
- Seek to understand your child's concerns and how they may differ from yours.
- Make room for them to speak, but don't pressure them to do so. Remember that sitting in silence with someone is a way of showing support and love.
- Be ready to end the conversation if saying more would dilute what has been said or you think your child cannot process anything else, while making it clear that you are always available to talk and answer questions. Say you'd like to check in again the next day.
- When you discuss concrete next steps or solutions to their difficulties, let them know that (depending on their age) they can play a role in their care. For example, having the final say on a therapist or psychiatrist can be a collaborative decision (if appropriate).
- If you believe your child is suicidal, don't delay. Call their pediatrician, a suicide hotline, or take them to the ER.

In this chapter, I've summarized the many ways that families can be touched by the effects of long Covid, and I hope that you have gained some insights and strategies to help you. But my biggest wish is that you've learned that being impacted by your loved one's illness is normal and perhaps even inevitable. You haven't faltered or failed but rather, your family, like all other families, is influenced by dynamics that develop around it.

When I was young, my grandparents lived in an old white craftsman-style house on what was left of their family farm. At the bottom of a hill behind the house sat a tiny pond and I would often go there, when I felt particularly grown up, to try and skip rocks. I loved to watch as the stones bounced across the surface and ripples on the water spread and multiplied and interconnected, causing waves on the far side of the pond. I've come to think of Covid, in many ways, as a skipping rock, sending out ripples in people's lives, as one change leads to many. Nowhere is this more evident than in long Covid, where the ripples just keep on going, and especially in families, where the effects of Covid-19 reverberate and impact not just one person but many. I'm hopeful that though things may be difficult for you and your family, this connection, and interconnection, can be a strength, and that you can help and support one another through this together.

Epilogue

It was the best of times, it was the worst of times..." Recently, this opening line of contrasts from Charles Dickens's *A Tale of Two Cities* has been reverberating in my head as I've come close to the end of writing this book. Over the last couple of years, I've witnessed the way that wildly different things can be true at the same time, that the best and worst can coexist, as I've watched the lives of long Covid survivors unfold. Their stories are personal, distinct, and unique, yet universal. I'll share two here, as I think they are emblematic of the way people can transition from surviving to thriving.

Just recently, at a support group, a few dozen patients and I heard some good news from Charlie, who has been a member of the group for more than a year. Strong, steady, and in his mid-fifties, he was critically ill with Covid-19 and a long and complex hospitalization nearly killed him. He went blind in one eye, lost seventy pounds from his already lean frame, and, with the accompanying muscle wastage, the ability to walk. Though physical therapy worked wonders, he continues to live with the lingering effects of cognitive impairment and trauma, including terrifying nightmares that visit him at least a few nights a week, like ghosts from another Charles Dickens novel. Unlike many of his peers, he managed to return to work, and, with help and support from his administration, has held on to his teaching job with a vise-like grip as it brings him such meaning. If he was a good teacher before, he is a better one now, he says, more loving, more patient, and imbued with a clear purpose.

At the support group session, Charlie told us, through tears, that he had just been voted Teacher of the Year by his peers at his South Carolina elementary school. His fellow survivors cheered at his words. For him, and for them, who had all played such a vital role in Charlie's recovery, this news was a triumph. A vindication, a validation, and proof that "misfit toys"—as one of the group's members refers to them—can achieve and accomplish great and hard things. Charlie's life is no picnic, but he'll be the first to say he's thriving, not merely surviving.

In contrast, Melanie's story does not include awards, but I would give her one if I could. When she called me out of the blue a few months ago, I answered, thinking I would hear her cheerful voice, but, instead, she was sobbing. She told me she was scared and tired and just couldn't keep going anymore, but she didn't want to die. I listened, knowing how badly her life had careened off the rails, driven by a toxic cocktail of fatigue, cognitive impairment, and depression after Covid. A proud mother and grandmother, with a house with a tidy yard and a white picket fence, her life had once been well ordered and filled with visits with family and friends, but in recent days her mind had taken her to dark places. "I'm terrified," she told me. "I've been thinking about driving my car into a tree, fast, just to be done." She took a deep breath, and I breathed in, too, on the other end of the line. "I can't do it though. I don't want a permanent solution to a hopefully temporary problem."

We talked back and forth, looking for a different solution, one that didn't dismiss her pain and fear but gave her a chance for healing. By the end of the call, she had promised to summon her "better angels" and check herself into the behavioral health hospital to keep herself safe. To give herself time and space to think. Later, she told me it was the first thing she had ever done for herself.

A few weeks ago, Melanie texted me, as she often does. She was back home, sitting in her yard, and feeling hopeful, no longer suicidal, but connected with psychiatric support and cobbling together a plan to live more fully and cope more effectively, even if her long Covid symptoms never go away. "I have a list of things I can still do," she said, "and I want to do them all." Is she thriving? Maybe. She's no longer just surviving.

I've been in the trenches with long Covid patients since the start of the pandemic, and I want a cure for this syndrome, or at least game-changing treatments, as much as anyone. For thousands of investigators, clinicians, and patient advocates, this desire motivates and animates, gets us out of bed in the morning, and keeps us burning the midnight oil. This urgency is driving research and clinical trials, many seeking to find the specific mechanisms underlying long Covid, including viral persistence,[1] an immune system gone awry,[2] and the presence of countless tiny blood clots generated by severe inflammation.[3] For now, many of these trials are relatively small and frustratingly incomplete, and we all long for the day when they are larger and more definitive.

While we wait, there are steps to take. There is support to be found, rehabilitation-related approaches to embrace, new narratives to write, pathways of advocacy to walk down, and healing to lean in to.

This isn't as good as a cure. It is a beginning. A formula for a life of hope, improvement, overcoming, and value. In the meantime, I promise to keep listening to my patients, learn from them, stay the course with them, and follow them into their lives to help them as best I can now and into the future as we find more answers.

I wish you all the best on your journey through long Covid. To return to Dickens, may you find a spring of hope after a winter of despair.

Acknowledgments

As a boy in the early 1980s, I was an average but enthusiastic baseball player and, even more passionately, an avid collector of baseball cards. I bought them at the grocery store and, on occasion, at the local antique mall and, one very happy day—to my great surprise—I received a paper bag full of them in the mail, sent to me from Illinois by my grandfather, Harold Jackson. He loved rummage sales and he had hit the mother lode, scoring hundreds of baseball cards from the 1960s for just a few dollars—cards of sluggers like Mickey Mantle and Harmon Killebrew, hitters like Al Kaline and Willie Mays and pitchers like Bob Gibson, Nolan Ryan, and Tom Seaver, and many more. I cherished these cards as my most prized possessions, showing them to my friends with pride, putting them in binders and staring at them for hours on end. I've been reflecting lately on my grandpa's loving gesture because it reminds me of the lavish generosity of so many people who have influenced, cared for, and challenged me and who, in so doing, have paved the way for the development of this book.

I'm particularly grateful for Lindsey Tate, my erstwhile editor and book coach. We had a phone call one rainy day in January to discuss what was a raw and embryonic idea and in a few short weeks we cemented a partnership and were off to the races. She is a gifted muse, a brilliant wordsmith, and far more than that, a good and faithful friend, and her lilting accent always reminds me of a peaceful English garden. She's generous, sincere, and authentic, and I'm particularly happy because I know that the connection we've built will remain for years and decades to come. I'm thankful, too, for my agent, Zoë Pagnamenta, whose expertise, gentle guidance, and superb instincts have been extraordinarily helpful and who, in her kind and reassuring way, has reminded me to keep calm and carry on as she's supported me in remembering that creating a book is a marathon and not a sprint. Finally, I'm deeply appreciative of my publisher, Tracy Behar, whose sage advice and active engagement has been crucial to the development of *Clearing the Fog*. I'll always be so delighted that I've had the ability to be supported by this trifecta of colleagues—thank you one and all.

Moving from the literary arena to the academic and clinical one, I feel fortunate and blessed to have learned under the steady and dynamic tutelage of one of the greatest critical care doctors and medical humanists in the world, my close friend, Dr. E. Wesley "Wes" Ely, who hired me to join his fledgling team (now known as the CIBS Center) more than twenty years ago. He's been a committed friend and mentor, a wise and vulnerable guide, and so many of the good things that have emerged in me as I care for patients and write their stories are directly attributable to his influence. I owe a similar debt to Dr. Mona Hopkins, a preeminent neuroscientist and an extraordinary person who taught me about the effects of illness on the brain and who was willing to sacrifice time and effort—again and again—to teach me about neuropsychology and, more crucially, about the impact in the lives of patients that a well-lived life of research can make. I would be more than a little remiss if I didn't mention my clinic partner, Dr. Carla Sevin. We jumped into the deep end together a decade ago and founded the ICU Recovery Center at Vanderbilt and, since that time, we've linked arms almost every Friday as we've cared for survivors of critical illness and Covid. She has stimulated my thinking about survival from illness in ways big and small and our patients are better as a result. Finally, I'm deeply grateful for my dear friends, psychologists Dr. Erin Hall and Dr. Megan Hosey, who from their posts at Geisinger Medical Center and Johns Hopkins Hospital have been two of my most ardent and thoughtful supporters since the start of the pandemic. Their knowledge of how to care for survivors of critical illness has been valuable, yes, but the far greater gift they bestowed on me has been their unwavering encouragement and support during the creation of *Clearing the Fog.* Thank you, friends, to all of you.

In the domain of work, I've been blessed to connect with Covid-19 survivors and long haulers since the very early days of the pandemic, made possible by a large and growing infrastructure that has allowed us to develop new programs, treatment paradigms, and research ideas, many of which have found their way into *Clearing the Fog.* How has this been possible and why does this infrastructure exist? I primarily credit my colleagues Amy Kiehl and Erin Collar. A little more than a decade ago, I made one of the best decisions of my life. Standing underneath a boat hanging from the ceiling of the Newport, Rhode Island, airport, I offered a job to Amy over the phone and two weeks later she became the master architect of what we've called our Long-Term Follow-Up Core at the CIBS Center. Not long after, Erin arrived, with attention to detail, fastidiousness, and a relatable Midwestern way (along with a dislike of the 1980s rock ballads that I constantly sing). Their partnership has resulted in the seamless creation of support groups, educational and social work–related programs and in the implementation and oversight of more than seventy-five studies, including thirty-four that are active, and many of which have focused on individuals with long Covid. They lovingly and expertly lead a team of about ten coordinators and, to put it bluntly, they get things done, ensuring that the research we are stewarded to deliver is done in a way that honors our patients and produces results that promise to impact the lives of others, even people we never meet. I want to thank them and let them know that I appreciate them so much.

Many coaches, mentors, friends, and a therapist or two have contributed to my life in ways that informed my desire to write *Clearing the Fog* and bolstered me during its development. In the last year, I lost two towering figures in my life: my high school football coach, Bob Knight, who died more quickly of cancer than any of us thought he would, and my college professor and mentor, Dr. Walt Russell, a brilliant scholar who succumbed to Alzheimer's dementia. I was able to talk to my old coach a few weeks before he left the world to thank him for two-a-day practices that felt like they would never end, for the way he prodded and provoked and inspired me, reminding me that I could do hard things that transcended any gridiron. I was less fortunate with my beloved teacher but if I was given the chance, I would have thanked him for his inestimable contributions to my life, for his contagious faith, for modeling a life of playful joy and intentional engagement with others and for being, at different times and places, a lifeline for me as I tried to figure out both who I was and what path I was destined to chart. His vulnerability, popular now, but hardly in vogue during the days that I saw him display it, was a way of life that I've tried imperfectly to embrace. I would also like to thank the psychologist whose warmth, compassion, and rigorous adherence to empirically guided treatment helped me immeasurably during the many hard days that I grappled with the impact of obsessive-compulsive disorder. I've certainly thanked her before for saving my life by inviting me to face my fears and to dust myself off and do it again but I'm not sure I can express my gratitude often enough.

For the last several years, in a season that has been filled with more isolation than usual in the context of the pandemic, I've been heartened and encouraged by a cadre of old high school classmates, connecting in a texting group at least every week and sometimes almost every day. I've been busy engaging old happy memories and sharing new ones with Amy, Andrea, Bob, Deb, Don, Flip, Lisa, Lisa, Mike, and Scott. Their warmth and affirmation have often carried me on challenging days, and I'm grateful. I'm so happy, too, to have many friends who have encouraged me, checked on me, and sometimes, even offered me a bit of tough love as they've nudged me toward the finish line on days that it felt like *Clearing the Fog* would never quite be completed— thanks, Ali, CD, Don, and Mike.

I was recently eating breakfast in Chicago, and as I surveyed the restaurant, I noticed one of the patients featured in *Clearing the Fog* sitting at a table a few feet from me. What a small world! We had a brief but lovely reunion and I was reminded, again, of how generous she was in allowing me to tell her story. I emphasize this because at the end of the day, *Clearing the Fog* is about people—real people whose bravery, grit, and resilience is inspiring and compelling. I'll always be grateful for the way Covid survivors—often in support groups, sometimes in the clinic, and sometimes in the context of consultations—have invited me into their lives, allowing me to learn about their challenges and triumphs and to join them on winding and sometimes, very hard, journeys. They are the heroes of this book and I pray daily that we would all be as kind and generous as they and that the lessons they've shared with me would ultimately contribute to the healing and betterment of others.

I want to thank my family and, in particular, my wife, Michelle. She and I met in 1991, and, since our first date at Fat Matt's Rib Shack in Atlanta, my life has been transformed by her joie de vivre, by the depth of her love for me and our children, and by the goodness that she radiates to all who come into her orbit. She has been my greatest supporter, spurring me on toward bigger and better horizons than I could imagine, including the writing of *Clearing the Fog,* and being a sojourner with her in this life is a high privilege. I'm also profoundly appreciative of my children—Carson, Colin, and Caroline—who have allowed me to spend time writing that I would otherwise have spent with them—loving this crew, learning from them, and cheering them on as they mature into wondrous and winsome humans is one of my greatest privileges and a source of such joy. My parents, Jim and Kathy Jackson, have sacrificially urged me to pursue goals and dreams, whatever they might be, since I was, as the saying goes, knee high to a grasshopper, and I honor them here. You could search far and wide and you would not find two finer people; I'm proud and humbled to be their son. In quiet, thoughtful, and unassuming ways, they have done so much for so many and a life of service, authentic and durable, is one of the gifts they've passed on to me—thank you for everything, Mom and Dad. I'm grateful, too, for my brother, Jon, five years younger than me, though I nonetheless aspire to be like him when I grow up and I appreciate his unfailing support.

Finally, I'm thankful for Jesus, the gentle Good Shepherd. For more than fifty years, He's walked with me through valleys, on joy-filled mountaintops, and everywhere in between. His yoke is easy, and His burden is light, and I owe Him a debt I can never repay.

Notes

Introduction

1. Davis, H. E., Assaf, G. S., McCorkell, L., Wei, H., Low, R. J., Re'em, Y., & Akrami, A. (2021). Characterizing long COVID in an international cohort: 7 months of symptoms and their impact. *EClinicalMedicine, 38,* 101019.

2. Chen, C., Haupert, S. R., Zimmermann, L., Shi, X., Fritsche, L. G., & Mukherjee, B. (2022). Global prevalence of post-coronavirus disease 2019 (COVID-19) condition or long covid: A meta-analysis and systematic review. *The Journal of Infectious Diseases.* https://doi.org/10.1093/infdis/jiac136

3. *Worldwide cancer data: World cancer research fund international.* WCRF International. (2022, April 14). Retrieved October 30, 2022, from https://www.wcrf.org/cancer-trends/worldwide-cancer-data/

4. Total population by country 2022. (n.d.). Retrieved October 30, 2022, from https://worldpopulationreview.com/countries

5. https://www.icudelirium.org

6. Kedor, C. et al. 2022. A prospective observational study of post-COVID-19 chronic fatigue syndrome following the first pandemic wave in Germany and biomarkers associated with symptom severity. *Nat. Commun.* 13, 5104

7. Groff D, Sun A, Ssentongo AE, et al. Short-term and Long-term Rates of Postacute Sequelae of SARS-CoV-2 Infection: A Systematic Review. *JAMA Netw Open.* 2021;4(10):e2128568. doi:10.1001/jamanetworkopen.2021.28568

8. Azoulay, E., Pochard, F., Kentish-Barnes, N., Chevret, S., Aboab, J., Adrie, C., Annane, D., Bleichner, G., Bollaert, P. E., Darmon, M., Fassier, T., Galliot, R., Garrouste-Orgeas, M., Goulenok, C., Goldgran-Toledano, D., Hayon, J., Jourdain, M., Kaidomar, M., Laplace, C., Larché, J., . . . FAMIREA Study Group (2005). Risk of post-traumatic stress symptoms in family members of intensive care unit patients. *American journal of respiratory and critical care medicine, 171*(9), 987–994. https://doi.org/10.1164/rccm.200409-1295OC

9. Johnson, C. C., Suchyta, M. R., Darowski, E. S., Collar, E. M., Kiehl, A. L., Van, J., Jackson, J. C., & Hopkins, R. O. (2019). Psychological Sequelae in Family Caregivers of Critically Ill Intensive Care Unit Patients. A Systematic Review. *Annals of the American Thoracic Society, 16*(7), 894–909. https://doi.org/10.1513/AnnalsATS.201808-540SR

Chapter 1

1. *Post-covid care centers.* Survivor Corps. (n.d.). Retrieved October 30, 2022, from https://www.survivorcorps.com/pccc
2. Roghanizad, M. M., & Bohns, V. K. (2017). Ask in person: You're less persuasive than you think over email. *Journal of Experimental Social Psychology, 69,* 223-226.

Chapter 2

1. Sarker, A., & Ge, Y. (2021). Mining long-COVID symptoms from Reddit: characterizing post-COVID syndrome from patient reports. *JAMIA open, 4*(3), ooab075
2. Guo, P., Benito Ballesteros, A., Yeung, S. P., Liu, R., Saha, A., Curtis, L., Kaser, M., Haggard, M. P., & Cheke, L. G. (2022). COVCOG 2: Cognitive and Memory Deficits in Long COVID: A Second Publication From the COVID and Cognition Study. Frontiers in aging neuroscience, 14, 804937. https://doi.org/10.3389/fnagi.2022.804937
3. Guo, P., Benito Ballesteros, A., Yeung, S. P., Liu, R., Saha, A., Curtis, L., Kaser, M., Haggard, M. P., & Cheke, L. G. (2022). COVCOG 1: Factors Predicting Physical, Neurological and Cognitive Symptoms in Long COVID in a Community Sample. A First Publication From the COVID and Cognition Study. Frontiers in aging neuroscience, 14, 804922. https://doi.org/10.3389/fnagi.2022.804922
4. Douaud, G., Lee, S., Alfaro-Almagro, F., Arthofer, C., Wang, C., McCarthy, P., . . . & Smith, S. M. (2022). SARS-CoV-2 is associated with changes in brain structure in UK Biobank. *Nature, 604*(7907), 697-707
5. Menon, D., Hampshire, A., Chatfield, D., Manktelow, A., Jolly, A., Trender, W., . . . & COVID, C. N. (2022). Multivariate profile and acute-phase correlates of cognitive deficits in a COVID-19 hospitalised cohort. *EClinicalMedicine, 47,* 101417.
6. Hampshire, A., Chatfield, D. A., Jolly, A., Trender, W., Hellyer, P. J., Del Giovane, M., . . . & Menon, D. K. (2022). Multivariate profile and acute-phase correlates of cognitive deficits in a COVID-19 hospitalised cohort. *EClinical Medicine, 47,* 101417.
7. Hampshire, A., Chatfield, D. A., Jolly, A., Trender, W., Hellyer, P. J., Del Giovane, M., . . . & Menon, D. K. (2022). Multivariate profile and acute-phase correlates of cognitive deficits in a COVID-19 hospitalised cohort. *EClinical Medicine, 47,* 101417.
8. Figueriedo, C.P., Barros-Aragão, F.G.Q., Neris, R.L.S. *et al.* Zika virus replicates in adult human brain tissue and impairs synapses and memory in mice. *Nat Commun* 10, 3890 (2019). https://doi.org/10.1038/s41467-019-11866-7
9. Chertow, D.S. Understanding long-term effects of Ebola virus disease. *Nat Med* 25, 714–715 (2019). https://doi.org/10.1038/s41591-019-0444-0
10. Pinnock, F., Rich, J., Vasquez, B., Wiegand, M., Patcai, J., Troyer, A., & Murphy, K. (2022). Neurocognitive Outcome Following Recovery from Severe Acute Respiratory Syndrome — Coronavirus-1 (SARS-CoV-1). *Journal of the International Neuropsychological Society, 28*(9), 891-901. doi:10.1017/S1355617721001107

11. Choutka, J., Jansari, V., Hornig, M. & Iwasaki, A. (2022). Unexplained post-acute infection syndromes. *Nat. Med.* 28, 911 -923.

12. Davis, H.E., McCorkell, L., Vogel, J.M. *et al.* (2023) Long COVID: major findings, mechanisms and recommendations. *Nat Rev Microbiol* 21, 133-146.

13. Monje and Iwasaki, The neurobiology of long COVID, Neuron (2022), https://doi.org/10.1016/j.neuron.2022.10.006

14. American Psychiatric Association. (2022). *Diagnostic and statistical manual of mental disorders* (5th ed., text rev.). https://doi.org/10.1176/appi.books. 9780890425787

15. Ferrucci, R., Dini, M., Rosci, C., Capozza, A., Groppo, E., Reitano, M. R., ... & Priori, A. (2022). One-year cognitive follow-up of COVID-19 hospitalized patients. *European Journal of Neurology*

16. Dini, M., Groppo, E., Chiara, R., Reitano, M., Allocco, E., Brugnera, A., ... & Ferrucci, R. (2021). Prolonged cognitive deficits after COVID-19. *Journal of the Neurological Sciences, 429.*

17. Krishnan, K., Miller, A. K., Reiter, K., & Bonner-Jackson, A. (2022). Neurocognitive profiles in patients with persisting cognitive symptoms associated with COVID-19. *Archives of Clinical Neuropsychology, 37*(4), 729-737.

18. Ferrucci, R., Dini, M., Groppo, E., Rosci, C., Reitano, M. R., Bai, F., ... & Priori, A. (2021). Long-lasting cognitive abnormalities after COVID-19. *Brain Sciences, 11*(2), 235.

19. Walshe, E. A., Ward McIntosh, C., Romer, D., & Winston, F. K. (2017). Executive Function Capacities, Negative Driving Behavior and Crashes in Young Drivers. *International journal of environmental research and public health, 14*(11), 1314. https://doi.org/10.3390/ijerph14111314

20. Pope, C. N., Bell, T. R., & Stavrinos, D. (2017). Mechanisms behind distracted driving behavior: The role of age and executive function in the engagement of distracted driving. *Accident; analysis and prevention, 98,* 123–129. https://doi.org/10.1016/j.aap.2016.09.030

21. Ikezaki, H., Hashimoto, M., Ishikawa, T., Fukuhara, R., Tanaka, H., Yuki, S., ... & Takebayashi, M. (2020). Relationship between executive dysfunction and neuropsychiatric symptoms and impaired instrumental activities of daily living among patients with very mild Alzheimer's disease. *International Journal of Geriatric Psychiatry, 35*(8), 877-887.

22. Spinella, M., Yang, B., & Lester, D. (2007). Development of the executive personal finance scale. *International Journal of Neuroscience, 117*(3), 301-313.

23. Boyle, P. A., Yu, L., Wilson, R. S., Segawa, E., Buchman, A. S., & Bennett, D. A. (2013). Cognitive decline impairs financial and health literacy among community-based older persons without dementia. *Psychology and aging, 28*(3), 614. Is health literacy the same as this?

24. Jackson, J. C., Girard, T. D., Gordon, S. M., Thompson, J. L., Shintani, A. K., Thomason, J. W., Pun, B. T., Canonico, A. E., Dunn, J. G., Bernard, G. R., Dittus, R. S., & Ely, E. W. (2010). Long-term cognitive and psychological outcomes in the awakening and breathing controlled trial. *American journal of respiratory and critical care medicine, 182*(2), 183–191. https://doi.org/10.1164 /rccm.200903-0442OC

Chapter 3

1. Hopkins, R. O., Weaver, L. K., Pope, D., Orme, J. F., Bigler, E. D., & Larson-LOHR, V. (1999). Neuropsychological sequelae and impaired health status in survivors of severe acute respiratory distress syndrome. *American journal of respiratory and critical care medicine, 160*(1), 50–56. https://doi.org/10.1164/ajrccm.160.1.9708059

2. Pandharipande, P. P., Girard, T. D., Jackson, J. C., Morandi, A., Thompson, J. L., Pun, B. T., ... & Ely, E. W. (2013). Long-term cognitive impairment after critical illness. *New England Journal of Medicine, 369*(14), 1306-1316.

3. Syed Alwi, Syarifah Maisarah MHSC1; Narayanan, Vairavan MHSC2; Che Din, Normah PhD3; Mohd Taib, Nur Aishah MD4. Cognitive Rehabilitation Programs for Survivors of Breast Cancer Treated With Chemotherapy: A Systematic Review. Rehabilitation Oncology: October 2021—Volume 39—Issue 4—p 155-167 doi: 10.1097/01.REO.0000000000000268

4. Chen, M. H., Chiaravalloti, N. D., & DeLuca, J. (2021). Neurological update: Cognitive rehabilitation in multiple sclerosis. *Journal of Neurology, 268*(12), 4908-4914.

5. Twamley, E. W., Thomas, K. R., Gregory, A. M., Jak, A. J., Bondi, M. W., Delis, D. C., & Lohr, J. B. (2015). CogSMART Compensatory Cognitive Training for Traumatic Brain Injury: Effects Over 1 Year. *The Journal of head trauma rehabilitation, 30*(6), 391–401. https://doi.org/10.1097/HTR.0000000000000076

6. Jackson, J. C., & Ely, E. W. (2013). Cognitive impairment after critical illness: etiologies, risk factors, and future directions. *Seminars in respiratory and critical care medicine, 34*(2), 216–222. https://doi.org/10.1055/s-0033-1342984

7. Robertson, I. H. (1996). *Goal management training: A clinical manual.* Cambridge: PsyConsult.

8. Levine, B., Stamenova, V. (2018). Goal Management Training. In: Kreutzer, J.S., DeLuca, J., Caplan, B. (eds) Encyclopedia of Clinical Neuropsychology. Springer, Cham. https://doi.org/10.1007/978-3-319-57111-9_9048

9. https://www.akiliinteractive.com/news-collection/akili-collaborates-with-weill-cornell-medicine-newyork-presbyterian-hospital-and-vanderbilt-university-medical-center-to-study-digital-therapeutic-akl-t01-as-treatment-for-covid-brain-fog

10. https://www.akiliinteractive.com/news-collection/akili-announces-endeavortm-attention-treatment-is-now-available-for-children-with-attention-deficit-hyperactivity-disorder-adhd-al3pw

11. Mahncke, H. W., Bronstone, A., & Merzenich, M. M. (2006). Brain plasticity and functional losses in the aged: scientific bases for a novel intervention. *Progress in brain research, 157,* 81–109. https://doi.org/10.1016/S0079-6123(06)57006-2

Chapter 4

1. Taquet, M., Geddes, J. R., Husain, M., Luciano, S., & Harrison, P. J. (2021). 6-month neurological and psychiatric outcomes in 236 379 survivors of COVID-19: a retrospective cohort study using electronic health records. *The Lancet Psychiatry, 8*(5), 416-427

2. Perlis, R. H., Ognyanova, K., Santillana, M., Baum, M. A., Lazer, D., Druckman, J., & Della Volpe, J. (2021). Association of acute symptoms of COVID-19 and symptoms of depression in adults. *JAMA network open, 4*(3), e213223-e213223.

3. Janiri, D., Carfì, A., Kotzalidis, G. D., Bernabei, R., Landi, F., Sani, G.,...& Post-Acute Care Study Group. (2021). Posttraumatic stress disorder in patients after severe COVID-19 infection. *JAMA psychiatry, 78*(5), 567-569.

4. Han, Q., Zheng, B., Daines, L., & Sheikh, A. (2022). Long-Term Sequelae of COVID-19: A Systematic Review and Meta-Analysis of One-Year Follow-Up Studies on Post-COVID Symptoms. *Pathogens (Basel, Switzerland), 11*(2), 269

5. Dar, S. A., Dar, M. M., Sheikh, S., Haq, I., Azad, A., Mushtaq, M., Shah, N. N., & Wani, Z. A. (2021). Psychiatric comorbidities among COVID-19 survivors in North India: A cross-sectional study. *Journal of education and health promotion, 10*, 309. https://doi.org/10.4103/jehp.jehp_119_21

6. https://time.com/6140256/ocd-covid-19-anxiety/

7. https://www.cancer.gov/publications/dictionaries/cancer-terms/def/watchful-waiting

Chapter 5

1. https://www.nami.org/mhstats

2. Shapiro, F. (1995). Eye movement desensitization and reprocessing. Use in PTSD: Schrader, C., & Ross, A. (2021). A Review of PTSD and Current Treatment Strategies. *Missouri medicine, 118*(6), 546–551.

3. De Lorenzo, R., Conte, C., Lanzani, C., Benedetti, F., Roveri, L., Mazza, M. G., Brioni, E., Giacalone, G., Canti, V., Sofia, V., D'Amico, M., Di Napoli, D., Ambrosio, A., Scarpellini, P., Castagna, A., Landoni, G., Zangrillo, A., Bosi, E., Tresoldi, M., Ciceri, F.,...Rovere-Querini, P. (2020). Residual clinical damage after COVID-19: A retrospective and prospective observational cohort study. *PloS one, 15*(10), e0239570. https://doi.org/10.1371/journal.pone.0239570

4. Schou, T. M., Joca, S., Wegener, G., & Bay-Richter, C. (2021). Psychiatric and neuropsychiatric sequelae of COVID-19 — A systematic review. *Brain, behavior, and immunity, 97*, 328–348. https://doi.org/10.1016/j.bbi.2021.07.018

5. Drew, B. L. (2001). Self-harm behavior and no-suicide contracting in psychiatric inpatient settings. *Archives of psychiatric nursing, 15*(3), 99-106.

Chapter 6

1. Lee, E. B., An, W., Levin, M. E., & Twohig, M. P. (2015). An initial meta-analysis of Acceptance and Commitment Therapy for treating substance use disorders. *Drug and alcohol dependence, 155*, 1–7. https://doi.org/10.1016/j.drugalcdep.2015.08.004

2. Yıldız E. (2020). The effects of acceptance and commitment therapy in psychosis treatment: A systematic review of randomized controlled trials. *Perspectives in psychiatric care, 56*(1), 149–167. https://doi.org/10.1111/ppc.12396

3. Arch, J. J., Eifert, G. H., Davies, C., Plumb Vilardaga, J. C., Rose, R. D., & Craske, M. G. (2012). Randomized clinical trial of cognitive behavioral

therapy (CBT) versus acceptance and commitment therapy (ACT) for mixed anxiety disorders. *Journal of consulting and clinical psychology, 80*(5), 750–765. https://doi.org/10.1037/a0028310

4. Bai, Z., Luo, S., Zhang, L., Wu, S., & Chi, I. (2020). Acceptance and Commitment Therapy (ACT) to reduce depression: A systematic review and meta-analysis. *Journal of affective disorders, 260,* 728–737. https://doi.org/10.1016/j.jad.2019.09.040

5. Hughes, L. S., Clark, J., Colclough, J. A., Dale, E., & McMillan, D. (2017). Acceptance and Commitment Therapy (ACT) for Chronic Pain: A Systematic Review and Meta-Analyses. *The Clinical journal of pain, 33*(6), 552–568. https://doi.org/10.1097/AJP.0000000000000425

6. Fogelkvist, M., Gustafsson, S. A., Kjellin, L., & Parling, T. (2020). Acceptance and commitment therapy to reduce eating disorder symptoms and body image problems in patients with residual eating disorder symptoms: A randomized controlled trial. *Body image, 32,* 155–166. https://doi.org/10.1016/j.bodyim.2020.01.002

Chapter 7

1. Tedeschi, R. G., Park, C. L., & Calhoun, L. G. (Eds.). (1998). *Posttraumatic growth: Positive changes in the aftermath of crisis.* Routledge.

2. Wu, X., Kaminga, A. C., Dai, W., Deng, J., Wang, Z., Pan, X., & Liu, A. (2019). The prevalence of moderate-to-high posttraumatic growth: A systematic review and meta-analysis. *Journal of affective disorders, 243,* 408–415.

3. Tanyi, Z., Mirnics, Z., Ferenczi, A., Smohai, M., Mészáros, V., Kovács, D., ... & Kövi, Z. (2020). Cancer as a source of posttraumatic growth: A brief review. *Psychiatria Danubina, 32*(suppl. 4), 401–411.

4. Vishnevsky, T., Cann, A., Calhoun, L. G., Tedeschi, R. G., & Demakis, G. J. (2010). Gender differences in self-reported posttraumatic growth: A meta-analysis. *Psychology of women quarterly, 34*(1), 110–120.

5. Widows, M. R., Jacobsen, P. B., Booth-Jones, M., & Fields, K. K. (2005). Predictors of posttraumatic growth following bone marrow transplantation for cancer. *Health psychology, 24*(3), 266.

6. Carola, V., Vincenzo, C., Morale, C., Pelli, M., Rocco, M., & Nicolais, G. (2022). Psychological health in COVID-19 patients after discharge from an intensive care unit. *Frontiers in public health, 10,* 951136. https://doi.org/10.3389/fpubh.2022.951136

7. Adjorlolo, S., Adjorlolo, P., Andoh-Arthur, J., Ahiable, E. K., Kretchy, I. A., & Osafo, J. (2022). Post-Traumatic Growth and Resilience among Hospitalized COVID-19 Survivors: A Gendered Analysis. *International journal of environmental research and public health, 19*(16), 10014. https://doi.org/10.3390/ijerph191610014

8. https://crsreports.congress.gov/product/pdf/R/R44321

9. Canevello, A., Michels, V., & Hilaire, N. (2016). Supporting close others' growth after trauma: The role of responsiveness in romantic partners' mutual posttraumatic growth. *Psychological trauma: theory, research, practice, and policy, 8*(3), 334.

10. Jia, X., Liu, X., Ying, L., & Lin, C. (2017). Longitudinal Relationships between Social Support and Posttraumatic Growth among Adolescent Survivors of the Wenchuan Earthquake. *Frontiers in psychology, 8,* 1275. https://doi.org/10.3389/fpsyg.2017.01275

11. Cadell, S., Regehr, C., & Hemsworth, D. (2003). Factors contributing to posttraumatic growth: A proposed structural equation model. *American Journal of Orthopsychiatry, 73*(3), 279-287.
Schroevers, M. J., Helgeson, V. S., Sanderman, R., & Ranchor, A. V. (2010). Type of social support matters for prediction of posttraumatic growth among cancer survivors. *Psycho-Oncology, 19*(1), 46-53.

Chapter 8

1. Livia Tomova, Kimberly L. Wang, Todd Thompson, Gillian A. Matthews, Atsushi Takahashi, Kay M. Tye, Rebecca Saxe. Acute social isolation evokes midbrain craving responses similar to hunger. *Nature Neuroscience,* 2020; 23 (12): 1597 DOI: 10.1038/s41593-020-00742-z

2. Santini, Z. I., Jose, P. E., York Cornwell, E., Koyanagi, A., Nielsen, L., Hinrichsen, C., Meilstrup, C., Madsen, K. R., & Koushede, V. (2020). Social disconnectedness, perceived isolation, and symptoms of depression and anxiety among older Americans (NSHAP): a longitudinal mediation analysis. *The Lancet. Public health, 5*(1), e62–e70. https://doi.org/10.1016/S2468-2667(19)30230-0

3. Cacioppo, J. T., Hughes, M. E., Waite, L. J., Hawkley, L. C., & Thisted, R. A. (2006). Loneliness as a specific risk factor for depressive symptoms: cross-sectional and longitudinal analyses. *Psychology and aging, 21*(1), 140–151. https://doi.org/10.1037/0882-7974.21.1.140

4. Kelly, M. M., DeBeer, B. B., Chamberlin, E., Claudio, T., Duarte, B., Harris, J. I., . . . & Reilly, E. D. (2022). The effects of loneliness and psychological flexibility on veterans' substance use and physical and mental health functioning during the COVID-19 pandemic. *Journal of Contextual Behavioral Science.*

5. Calati, R., Ferrari, C., Brittner, M., Oasi, O., Olié, E., Carvalho, A. F., & Courtet, P. (2019). Suicidal thoughts and behaviors and social isolation: A narrative review of the literature. *Journal of affective disorders, 245,* 653–667. https://doi.org/10.1016/j.jad.2018.11.022

6. Christiansen, J., Qualter, P., Friis, K., Pedersen, S. S., Lund, R., Andersen, C. M., Bekker-Jeppesen, M., & Lasgaard, M. (2021). Associations of loneliness and social isolation with physical and mental health among adolescents and young adults. *Perspectives in public health, 141*(4), 226–236. https://doi.org/10.1177/17579139211016077.

7. Yang, Y. C., Li, T., & Ji, Y. (2013). Impact of social integration on metabolic functions: evidence from a nationally representative longitudinal study of US older adults. *BMC public health, 13,* 1210. https://doi.org/10.1186/1471-2458-13-1210

8. Yang, Y. C., Li, T., & Ji, Y. (2013). Impact of social integration on metabolic functions: evidence from a nationally representative longitudinal study of US older adults. *BMC public health, 13,* 1210. https://doi.org/10.1186/1471-2458-13-1210.

9. Elmacıoğlu, F., Emiroğlu, E., Ülker, M. T., Özyılmaz Kırcali, B., & Oruç, S. (2021). Evaluation of nutritional behaviour related to COVID-19. *Public health nutrition, 24*(3), 512–518. https://doi.org/10.1017/S1368980020004140

10. Valtorta, N. K., Kanaan, M., Gilbody, S., Ronzi, S., & Hanratty, B. (2016). Loneliness and social isolation as risk factors for coronary heart disease and stroke: systematic review and meta-analysis of longitudinal observational studies. *Heart (British Cardiac Society), 102*(13), 1009–1016. https://doi.org/10.1136/heartjnl-2015-308790

11. Cacioppo, J. T., Hawkley, L. C., Berntson, G. G., Ernst, J. M., Gibbs, A. C., Stickgold, R., & Hobson, J. A. (2002). Do lonely days invade the nights? Potential social modulation of sleep efficiency. *Psychological science, 13*(4), 384–387. https://doi.org/10.1111/1467-9280.00469

12. Alcaraz, K. I., Eddens, K. S., Blase, J. L., Diver, W. R., Patel, A. V., Teras, L. R., Stevens, V. L., Jacobs, E. J., & Gapstur, S. M. (2019). Social Isolation and Mortality in US Black and White Men and Women. *American journal of epidemiology, 188*(1), 102–109. https://doi.org/10.1093/aje/kwy231

13. Holt-Lunstad, J., Smith, T. B., Baker, M., Harris, T., & Stephenson, D. (2015). Loneliness and social isolation as risk factors for mortality: a meta-analytic review. *Perspectives on psychological science: a journal of the Association for Psychological Science, 10*(2), 227–237. https://doi.org/10.1177/1745691614568352

14. Shen, C., Rolls, E. T., Cheng, W., Kang, J., Dong, G., Xie, C., . . . & Feng, J. (2022). Associations of social isolation and loneliness with later dementia. *Neurology, 99*(2), e164–e175.

15. Shang, Y., Wu, W., Dove, A., Guo, J., Welmer, A. K., Rizzuto, D., . . . & Xu, W. (2022). Healthy Behaviors, Leisure Activities, and Social Network Prolong Disability-Free Survival in Older Adults With Diabetes. *The Journals of Gerontology: Series A.*

16. Seeman, T. E., & Syme, S. L. (1987). Social networks and coronary artery disease: a comparison of the structure and function of social relations as predictors of disease. *Psychosomatic medicine.*

17. Holt-Lunstad, J., Smith, T. B., & Layton, J. B. (2010). Social relationships and mortality risk: a meta-analytic review. *PLoS medicine, 7*(7), e1000316.

18. Siette, J., Dodds, L., Surian, D., Prgomet, M., Dunn, A., & Westbrook, J. (2022). Social Interactions and quality of life of residents in aged care facilities: A multi-methods study. *PLOS ONE, 17*(8). https://doi.org/10.1371/journal.pone.0273412

19. Kuczynski, A. M., Halvorson, M. A., Slater, L. R., & Kanter, J. W. (2021). The effect of social interaction quantity and quality on depressed mood and loneliness: A daily diary study. *Journal of Social and Personal Relationships, 39*(3), 734–756. https://doi.org/10.1177/02654075211045717

20. Sandstrom, G. M., & Dunn, E. W. (2014). Social Interactions and well-being. *Personality and Social Psychology Bulletin, 40*(7), 910–922. https://doi.org/10.1177/0146167214529799

21. Allen, K.-A., Kern, M. L., Rozek, C. S., McInerney, D. M., & Slavich, G. M. (2021). Belonging: A review of Conceptual Issues, an integrative framework,

and directions for future research. *Australian Journal of Psychology, 73*(1), 87–102. https://doi.org/10.1080/00049530.2021.1883409

22. Felix, C., Rosano, C., Zhu, X., Flatt, J. D., & Rosso, A. L. (2021). Greater social engagement and greater gray matter microstructural integrity in brain regions relevant to dementia. *The Journals of Gerontology: Series B, 76*(6), 1027-1035.

Chapter 9

1. https://www.washingtonpost.com/business/2021/12/09/long-covid-work -unemployed/
2. Annikakimc. (2021, July 27). *Some Americans with 'long covid' may qualify for Federal Disability Resources, Biden says.* CNBC. Retrieved October 29, 2022, from https://www.cnbc.com/2021/07/26/long-covid-biden-says-some-qualify -for-federal-disability-resources.html
3. (OCR), O. for C. R. (2021, August 11). *Guidance on "long covid" as a disability under the Ada, section.* HHS.gov. Retrieved October 29, 2022, from https://www.hhs.gov/civil-rights/for-providers/civil-rights-covid19/guidance -long-covid-disability/index.html
4. *How to write a resignation letter.* Harvard Business Review. (2022, October 19). Retrieved October 29, 2022, from https://hbr.org/2022/07/how-to-write -a-resignation-letter

Chapter 10

1. Jafary Manesh, H., Ranjbaran, M., Vakilian, K., Rezaei, K., Zand, K., & Tajik, R. (2014). Survey of levels of anxiety and depression in parents of children with chronic illness. *Iranian Journal of Psychiatric Nursing, 1*(4), 45-53.
2. Pakenham, K. I. PhD, Cox, S., PhD, The Effects of Parental Illness and Other Ill Family Members on the Adjustment of Children, *Annals of Behavioral Medicine,* Volume 48, Issue 3, December 2014, Pages 424–437, https://doi.org /10.1007/s12160-014-9622-y
3. Pan, Y. C., & Lin, Y. S. (2022). Systematic Review and Meta-Analysis of Prevalence of Depression Among Caregivers of Cancer Patients. *Frontiers in psychiatry, 13,* 817936. https://doi.org/10.3389/fpsyt.2022.817936
4. Alliance, B. F. C. (n.d.). *Caregiver statistics: Health, Technology, and caregiving resources.* Caregiver Statistics: Health, Technology, and Caregiving Resources—Family Caregiver Alliance. Retrieved October 31, 2022, from https://www.caregiver .org/resource/caregiver-statistics-health-technology-and-caregiving-resources/
5. Weitzenkamp, D. A., Gerhart, K. A., Charlifue, S. W., Whiteneck, G. G., & Savic, G. (1997). Spouses of spinal cord injury survivors: the added impact of caregiving. *Archives of physical medicine and rehabilitation, 78*(8), 822-827.
6. Azoulay, E., Pochard, F., Kentish-Barnes, N., Chevret, S., Aboab, J., Adrie, C., Annane, D., Bleichner, G., Bollaert, P. E., Darmon, M., Fassier, T., Galliot, R., Garrouste-Orgeas, M., Goulenok, C., Goldgran-Toledano, D., Hayon, J., Jourdain, M., Kaidomar, M., Laplace, C., Larché, J., . . . FAMIREA Study Group (2005). Risk of post-traumatic stress symptoms in family members of intensive care unit patients. *American journal of respiratory and critical care medicine, 171*(9), 987–994. https://doi.org/10.1164/rccm.200409-1295OC

7. Kornblith, A. B., Herr, H. W., Ofman, U. S., Scher, H. I., & Holland, J. C. (1994). Quality of life of patients with prostate cancer and their spouses. The value of a data base in clinical care. *Cancer, 73*(11), 2791-2802.

8. Karraker, A., & Latham, K. (2015). In Sickness and in Health? Physical Illness as a Risk Factor for Marital Dissolution in Later Life. *Journal of health and social behavior, 56*(3), 420–435.https://doi.org/10.1177/0022146515596354

9. Kirchhoff, A. C., Yi, J., Wright, J., Warner, E. L., & Smith, K. R. (2012). Marriage and divorce among young adult cancer survivors. *Journal of Cancer Survivorship, 6*(4), 441–450. https://doi.org/10.1007/s11764-012-0238-6

10. Glantz, M. J., Chamberlain, M. C., Liu, Q., Hsieh, C. C., Edwards, K. R., Van Horn, A., & Recht, L. (2009). Gender disparity in the rate of partner abandonment in patients with serious medical illness. *Cancer, 115*(22), 5237-5242.

11. Sylvester, S. V., Rusu, R., Chan, B., Bellows, M., O'Keefe, C., & Nicholson, S. (2022). Sex differences in sequelae from COVID-19 infection and in long COVID syndrome: a review. *Current Medical Research and Opinion, 38*(8), 1391-1399.

12. White, M. P., Alcock, I., Grellier, J., Wheeler, B. W., Hartig, T., Warber, S. L., ... & Fleming, L. E. (2019). Spending at least 120 minutes a week in nature is associated with good health and well-being. *Scientific reports, 9*(1), 1-11.

13. de Witte, M., Pinho, A. D. S., Stams, G. J., Moonen, X., Bos, A. E., & van Hooren, S. (2022). Music therapy for stress reduction: a systematic review and meta-analysis. *Health Psychology Review, 16*(1), 134-159.

14. Racine, N., McArthur, B. A., Cooke, J. E., Eirich, R., Zhu, J., & Madigan, S. (2021). Global prevalence of depressive and anxiety symptoms in children and adolescents during COVID-19: a meta-analysis. *JAMA pediatrics, 175*(11), 1142-1150.

15. Worsham, N. L., Compas, B. E., & Ey, S. (1997). Children's coping with parental illness. In *Handbook of children's coping* (pp. 195-213). Springer, Boston, MA.

16. Stein JA, Newcomb MD. Children's internalizing and externalizing behaviors and maternal health problems. *J. Pediatr. Psychol.* 1994; 19: 571–93.

17. Elliott, L., Thompson, K. A., & Fobian, A. D. (2020). A Systematic Review of Somatic Symptoms in Children With a Chronically Ill Family Member. *Psychosomatic medicine, 82*(4), 366–376. https://doi.org/10.1097/PSY .0000000000000799

18. Sieh, D. S., Meijer, A. M., Oort, F. J., Visser-Meily, J. M., & Van der Leij, D. A. (2010). Problem behavior in children of chronically ill parents: a meta-analysis. *Clinical child and family psychology review, 13*(4), 384–397. https://doi .org/10.1007/s10567-010-0074-z

19. Bell, M. F., Bayliss, D. M., Glauert, R., & Ohan, J. L. (2019). Developmental vulnerabilities in children of chronically ill parents: a population-based linked data study. *Journal of epidemiology and community health, 73*(5), 393–400. https:// doi.org/10.1136/jech-2018-210992

20. Van der Werf, H. M., Luttik, M., Francke, A. L., Roodbol, P. F., & Paans, W. (2019). Students growing up with a chronically ill family member; a survey on

experienced consequences, background characteristics, and risk factors. *BMC public health, 19*(1), 1486. https://doi.org/10.1186/s12889-019-7834-6

Epilogue

1. Buonsenso, D., Piazza, M., Boner, A. L., & Bellanti, J. A. (2022). Long COVID: A proposed hypothesis-driven model of viral persistence for the pathophysiology of the syndrome. *Allergy and asthma proceedings, 43*(3), 187–193. https://doi.org/10.2500/aap.2022.43.220018
2. Noval Rivas, M., Porritt, R. A., Cheng, M. H., Bahar, I., & Arditi, M. (2022). Multisystem Inflammatory Syndrome in Children and Long COVID: The SARS-CoV-2 Viral Superantigen Hypothesis. *Frontiers in immunology, 13*, 941009. https://doi.org/10.3389/fimmu.2022.941009
3. Helen Fogarty, Soracha E. Ward, Liam Townsend, Ellie Karampini, Stephanie Elliott, Niall Conlon, Jean Dunne, Rachel Kiersey, Aifric Naughton, Mary Gardiner, Mary Byrne, Colm Bergin, Jamie M. O'Sullivan, Ignacio Martin-Loeches, Parthiban Nadarajan, Ciaran Bannan, Patrick W. Mallon, Gerard F. Curley, Roger J. S. Preston, Aisling M. Rehill, Ross I. Baker, Cliona Ni Cheallaigh, James S. O'Donnell, Niamh O'Connell, Kevin Ryan, Dermot Kenny, Judicael Fazavana. Sustained VWF-ADAMTS-13 axis imbalance and endotheliopathy in long COVID syndrome is related to immune dysfunction. *Journal of Thrombosis and Haemostasis,* 2022; DOI: 10.1111/jth.15830

Index

About the Author

Dr. James "Jim" Jackson is an internationally renowned expert on long Covid and its effects on cognitive and mental health functioning. A licensed psychologist specializing in neuropsychology and cognitive rehabilitation, he completed his psychology residency at the Veteran's Affairs/Vanderbilt University School of Medicine Consortium while also receiving post-doctoral training in cognitive rehabilitation at the Oliver Zangwill Center in Ely, England. A pioneer in the investigation and treatment of Post–Intensive Care Syndrome (PICS), — a condition that impacts up to a third of survivors of critical illness — he is a research professor of Medicine and Psychiatry at Vanderbilt, where he is also the co-founder and director of Behavioral Health at the award-winning ICU Recovery Center, one of the first comprehensive clinical resources devoted to diagnosing and treating survivors of both mild and critical illness, including those who survived Covid-19. There, Dr. Jackson consults with patients and their families from around the world. Additionally, he serves as the director of Long-Term Outcomes at the Critical Illness, Brain Dysfunction, and Survivorship (CIBS) Center (icudelirium.org), a consortium focused on advancing knowledge, education, and models of care for people affected by acute and long-term brain dysfunction following wide ranging illnesses (from mild to severe). He and his team created the first psychologist-led long Covid support groups in the United States early in the pandemic and continue to offer multiple groups every week. An influential researcher engaged in numerous investigations into the neuropsychological features of long Covid and the effects of cognitive rehabilitation, he is the author of over 150 scientific papers on illness and cognitive impairment published in leading peer-reviewed biomedical journals including *New England Journal of Medicine* (NEJM), *The Lancet*, and *Journal of the American Medical Association*, (JAMA), as well as many book chapters and editorials. His research program has been funded by the Department of Defense, Department of Veteran's Affairs, and the National Institute of Health and highlighted in the pages of *The Atlantic, Newsweek, The New York Times, Scientific American, Time, The Wall Street Journal, The Washington Post*, and *Wired*, as well as on *CNN* and *PBS* among dozens of others. Originally from Kalamazoo, Michigan, Dr. Jackson resides in Nashville, Tennessee with his wife, three children, and their dogs, Olive, and Waffles. Visit his website at jamescjackson.com.